ANATOMY FOR

BACK BENDS

AND

TWISTS

RAY LONG, MD, FRCSC

bandha yoga publications

This book is intended as a reference volume only, not as a medical manual. It is not to be used in any manner for diagnosis or treatment of medical or surgical conditions. This book is also not intended to be a substitute for any treatment that may be or has been prescribed by your health care provider. If you suspect that you have a medical problem, consult your physician. Always, in your particular case, obtain medical clearance from your physician before beginning the practice of yoga or any other exercise program. Always practice yoga under the direct guidance and supervision of a qualified and experienced instructor. Working directly with a qualified yoga instructor can help to prevent injuries. The author, illustrators, editor, publisher and distributor specifically disclaim any responsibility or liability for injuries that may occur during the practice of yoga or any other exercise program.

Published by Bandha Yoga Publications
Plattsburgh, NY
www.bandhayoga.com

Distributed by Greenleaf Book Group LLC

For ordering information and bulk purchases, contact Bandha Yoga Publications.
info@bandhayoga.com
Phone: 518.578.3720

Design and composition by Greenleaf Book Group LLC
Cover design by Greenleaf Book Group LLC
Front and back cover illustrations by Kurt Long, BFA   www.kurtlong.net
Computer Graphics Technical Director: Chris Macivor
Sanskrit calligraphy and border painting: Stewart Thomas   www.palmstone.com
Editor: Eryn Kirkwood, MA, RYT   www.barrhavenyoga.com

ISBN 13: 978-1-60743-944-8

Part of the Tree Neutral® program, which offsets the number of trees consumed in the production and printing of this book by taking proactive steps, such as planting trees in direct proportion to the number of trees used: www.treeneutral.com

Printed in China on acid-free paper

10 11 12 13 14 15   10 9 8 7 6 5 4 3 2 1

First Edition

CONTENTS

INTRODUCTION

PRACTICING YOGA IS NOT NECESSARILY THE PATH OF LEAST RESISTANCE. AND although the Sanskrit word asana translates to mean "a comfortable, easy position," most yoga poses are neither comfortable nor easy. Working with them, however, makes daily life more comfortable and easy.

So why integrate Western science into the ancient art of Hatha Yoga? Because scientific techniques enable you to intelligently design your practice and give you confidence in your teaching. Hatha Yoga works with the body and Western science understands how the body works.

For example, suppose you want to deepen a backbend such as Urdhva Dhanurasana. Knowledge of anatomy, biomechanics, and physiology enable you to predictably do this. Or if you're a teacher and a student comes to you with lower back discomfort in Camel Pose, you can use the abdominal "air bag" effect discussed in this book and often address the problem quickly and easily. Similarly, if you wish to deepen twists for yourself or your students, design your practice to involve physiological techniques such as facilitated stretching that will release and lengthen the muscles that inhibit turning the trunk. Many of these solutions would not be obvious, or would even be counterintuitive, unless you knew how to apply scientific principles to yoga. This book explains these techniques in detail, with their practical application for backbends and twists.

Spare no effort in searching out areas of resistance in your yoga poses. If your body is stiff, use the physiological techniques described in the Mat Companion series to lengthen muscles, break through barriers, and gain flexibility. If your body is flexible, then work with the bandhas described here to increase your strength.

Painter and sculptor George Braque once said, "Art disturbs, science reassures." The idea is that art takes one out of a comfort zone and into new experiences. Science provides grounding and stability. Yoga poses are like physical sculptures that take you out of your comfort zone. Scientific techniques are the sculpting tools that allow you to do this with intelligence and precision.

HOW TO USE THIS BOOK

Practicing yoga is like passing through a series of doors, with each door revealing new possibilities in the poses. The key to unlocking the first door is understanding the joint positions. This understanding can be used to identify the muscles that create the form of the pose and those that stretch. The key to positioning the joints is engaging the correct muscles. This begins with the prime movers. Engage the prime movers and the bones will align. The key to deepening the asanas is using your understanding of physiology to lengthen the muscles that stretch in the pose. Focus on these keys and the postures will automatically fall into place and manifest the beneficial effects of yoga. These include improved flexibility, heightened awareness, a sense of well-being, and deep relaxation.

The Mat Companion series is a set of modular books. Each book focuses on a specific pose category and contains the following:

- **The Key Concepts:** a description of biomechanical and physiological principles with applications for specific poses.
- **The Bandha Yoga Codex:** a simple five-step process that can be used to improve your flexibility, strength, and precision in the asanas.
- **The Pose Section:** a detailed description of the individual postures.
- **Movement Index:** explanations of body movement and tables listing the muscles associated with each movement.
- **Anatomy Index:** a visual listing of bones, ligaments, and muscles (showing the origins, insertions, and actions of each).
- **Glossary of Terms**
- **Sanskrit Pronunciation and Pose Index**
- **English Pose Index**

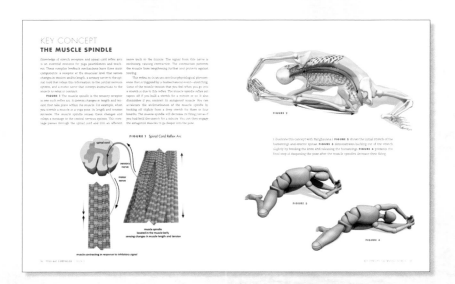

FIGURE 1 The Key Concepts show you how to apply biomechanics and physiology to your poses. Read this section first and return here often to refresh your knowledge.

FIGURE 2 The opening page for each pose illustrates the basic joint actions and positions of the body for that particular asana. Sanskrit and English names are provided for each posture. Use this page to assist you in learning the basic form of the pose and other concise details.

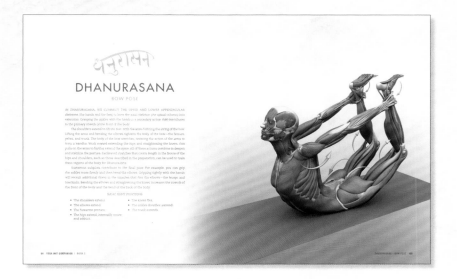

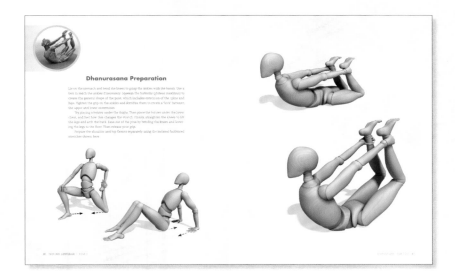

FIGURE 3 Use the preparatory section as a guide for how to enter the pose. If you are new to yoga or feel a bit stiff, use one of these modifications for your practice. In general, the preparatory poses affect the same muscle groups as the final asana. You will benefit from the pose no matter which variation you practice.

FIGURE 4 Each pose comes with a series of steps for engaging the muscles that position the joints, concluding with a summary of the muscles that stretch. Muscles that contract are colored different shades of blue (with the prime movers deep blue), and those that stretch are red. Use the pose section to master the anatomy of any given asana.

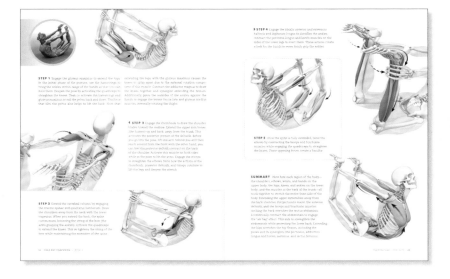

LOCATING THE
FOCUS OF A POSE

As we go through our day, we are always thinking about something—work, relationships, problems we're faced with. Practicing yoga draws the attention away from that "something" for a period of time and produces a cognitive shift. When we return to our activities of daily living, our perspective has changed. The affect of whatever was drawing our attention is often transformed.

All meditative and yogic practices contain an element of focus. The Sanskrit name for this is drishti. The location can be the breath, a part of the body, a bandha, or even a place on the wall where you focus your gaze. Hatha Yoga is a particularly powerful method for attaining a meditative state. In this practice, the body is the vehicle through which physical points of focus evoke mental transformations.

Triangulation is one means of locating focal points in the asanas. It is a technique used by film makers to draw attention to a character. An example might be two persons conspiring to affect a third. The third character then reacts, eliciting a counter-response and so on. This keeps the story moving. The process is called triangulation because each character forms a vertex of the triangle.

You can use triangulation in yoga poses. For example, in the forward bend Paschimottanasana, contract the psoas to flex the hips and tilt the pelvis forward, drawing the origin of the hamstrings back. Then contract the quadriceps to extend the knees and move the hamstrings' insertion on the lower leg. The pelvis pulls the hamstrings from one end, while the tibia pulls the muscle from the other. This creates a focal point on the hamstrings, which react by stretching.

Keep the story moving by changing the focal point. For example, in the same pose, bring your focus to the arms by contracting the biceps to flex the elbows. At the same time, engage the abdominals to flex the trunk. These two actions (or characters) conspire to lengthen the erector spinae of the back.

Moving through the postures stimulates the release of neurotransmitters called endorphins. These molecules interact with the same receptors in the brain as pain medications such as morphine, producing a sense of well-being and comfort. By incorporating precise scientific knowledge into your practice, you can augment the release of endorphins and amplify the cognitive shift produced by meditative focus.

Place your drishti on the muscle groups that create the form of the pose. In this manner you will improve the asanas and your meditative state. The result is a positive feedback loop. The biomechanics give a functional point of focus within the poses. The poses themselves evoke chemical changes that accentuate and increase the duration of the meditative state of mind.

KEY
CONCEPTS

KEY CONCEPT

AGONIST/ANTAGONIST RELATIONSHIPS: RECIPROCAL INHIBITION

Agonist/antagonist relationships form biomechanical and physiological focal points throughout the body in yoga poses. The angles and positions of the joints create the form of a pose. Agonist muscles contract to decrease the angle of the joint, while on the other side of the joint, the antagonist muscle stretches and the angle increases. Understanding this relationship is essential to sculpting any given pose.

Once you have identified the muscle groups surrounding each of the major joints, focus on contracting specific muscles to create and refine the form of the pose. Move your focus around the body, activating the agonist muscles to biomechanically triangulate their antagonists (as described in the section entitled Locating the Focus of a Pose). Contracting a muscle moves its origin and insertion closer to one another. The corresponding origin and insertion of that muscle's antagonist move farther apart, lengthening the muscle.

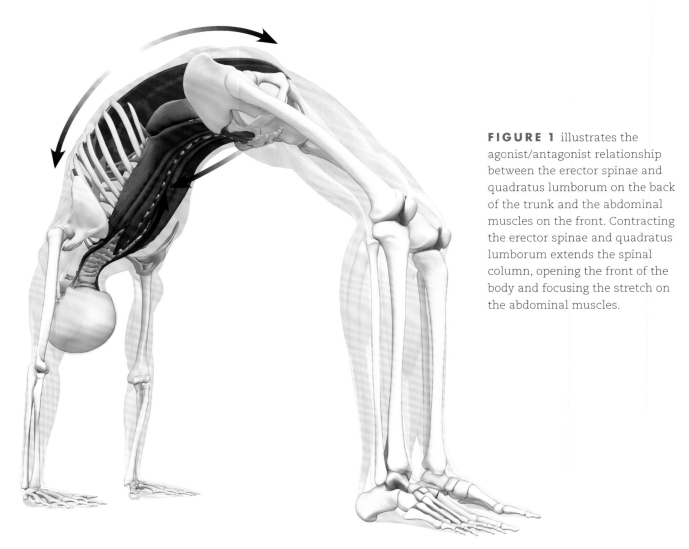

FIGURE 1 illustrates the agonist/antagonist relationship between the erector spinae and quadratus lumborum on the back of the trunk and the abdominal muscles on the front. Contracting the erector spinae and quadratus lumborum extends the spinal column, opening the front of the body and focusing the stretch on the abdominal muscles.

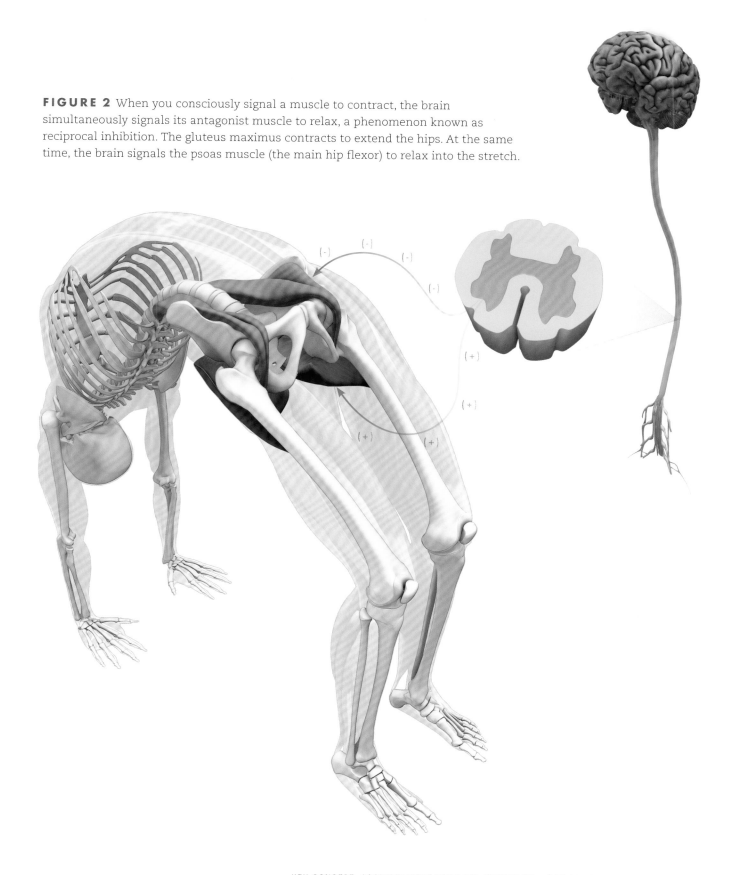

FIGURE 2 When you consciously signal a muscle to contract, the brain simultaneously signals its antagonist muscle to relax, a phenomenon known as reciprocal inhibition. The gluteus maximus contracts to extend the hips. At the same time, the brain signals the psoas muscle (the main hip flexor) to relax into the stretch.

FIGURE 3 illustrates another agonist/antagonist relationship for the hip joint. In this case, the hamstrings extend the hip. We typically think of the hamstrings as flexors of the knee; however, in Urdhva Dhanurasana the feet are fixed on the mat. Attempting to draw the feet towards the hands contracts the hamstrings and aids to extend the hips. This triangulates and focuses the stretch on the psoas and its synergists (the rectus femoris, pectineus, and adductors longus and brevis).

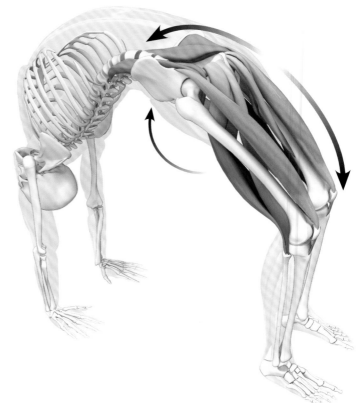

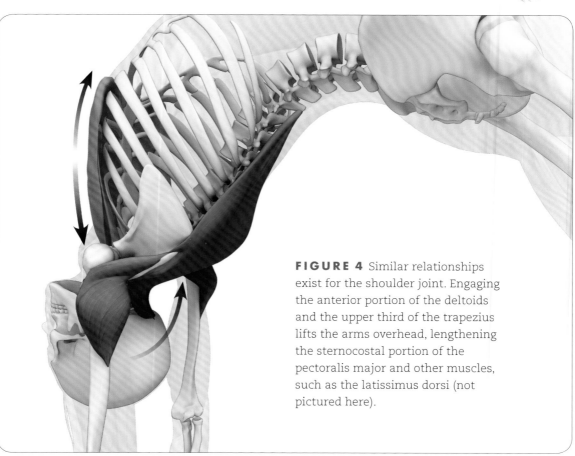

FIGURE 4 Similar relationships exist for the shoulder joint. Engaging the anterior portion of the deltoids and the upper third of the trapezius lifts the arms overhead, lengthening the sternocostal portion of the pectoralis major and other muscles, such as the latissimus dorsi (not pictured here).

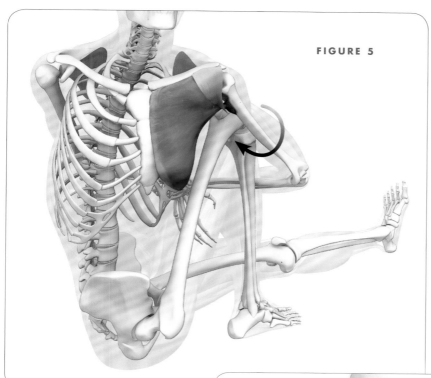

FIGURE 5

The pectoralis major, anterior portion of the deltoid, and subscapularis muscles internally rotate the humerus (**FIGURE 5**). This focuses the stretch on the infraspinatus, teres minor, and posterior portion of the deltoid in poses such as Marichyasana III (**FIGURE 6**).

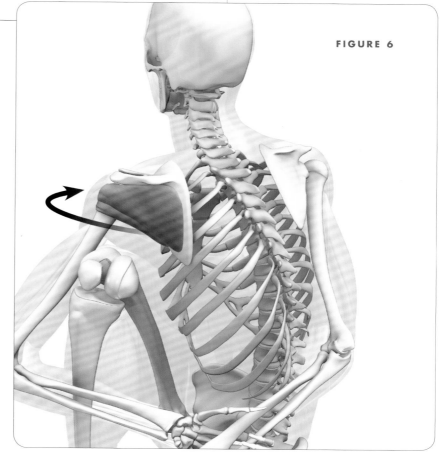

FIGURE 6

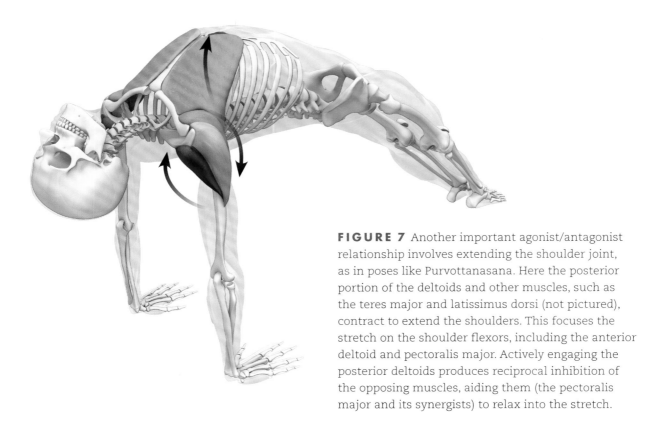

FIGURE 7 Another important agonist/antagonist relationship involves extending the shoulder joint, as in poses like Purvottanasana. Here the posterior portion of the deltoids and other muscles, such as the teres major and latissimus dorsi (not pictured), contract to extend the shoulders. This focuses the stretch on the shoulder flexors, including the anterior deltoid and pectoralis major. Actively engaging the posterior deltoids produces reciprocal inhibition of the opposing muscles, aiding them (the pectoralis major and its synergists) to relax into the stretch.

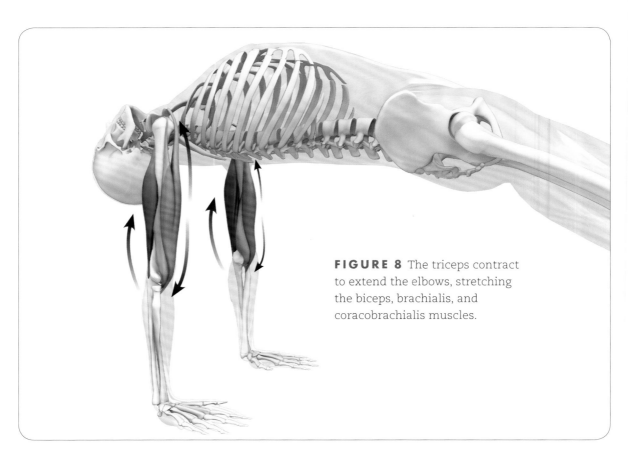

FIGURE 8 The triceps contract to extend the elbows, stretching the biceps, brachialis, and coracobrachialis muscles.

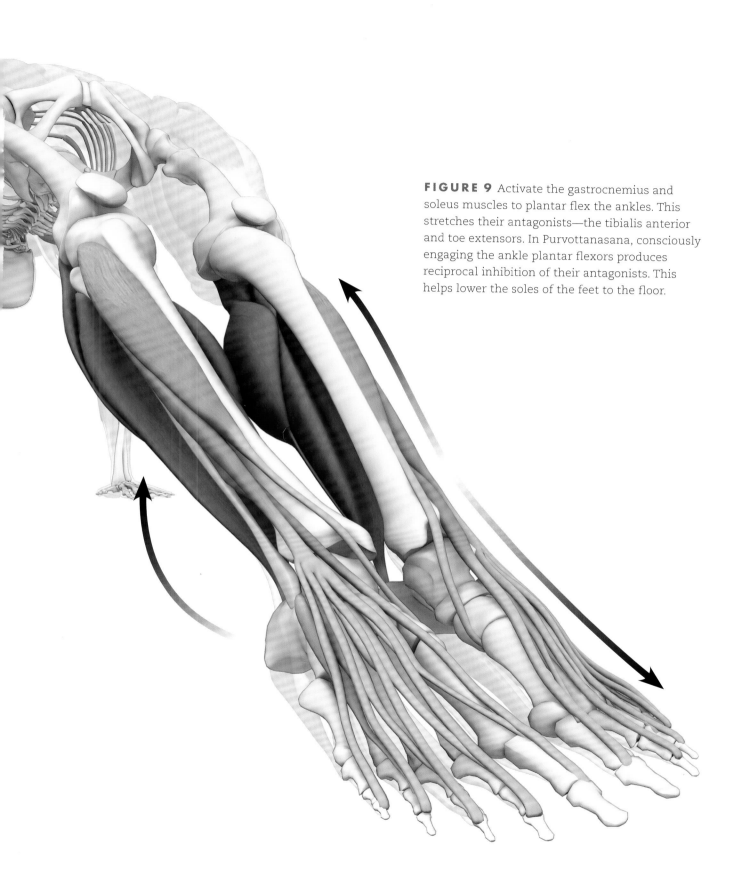

FIGURE 9 Activate the gastrocnemius and soleus muscles to plantar flex the ankles. This stretches their antagonists—the tibialis anterior and toe extensors. In Purvottanasana, consciously engaging the ankle plantar flexors produces reciprocal inhibition of their antagonists. This helps lower the soles of the feet to the floor.

KEY CONCEPT
KEY MUSCLE ISOLATIONS

Creating focal points in yoga poses involves engaging the muscle groups that produce the form of the pose. This automatically aligns the bones. Because it is not always obvious how to isolate a particular agonist muscle, we provide some cues for this here. Use these cues (and develop your own) to improve your practice and teaching.

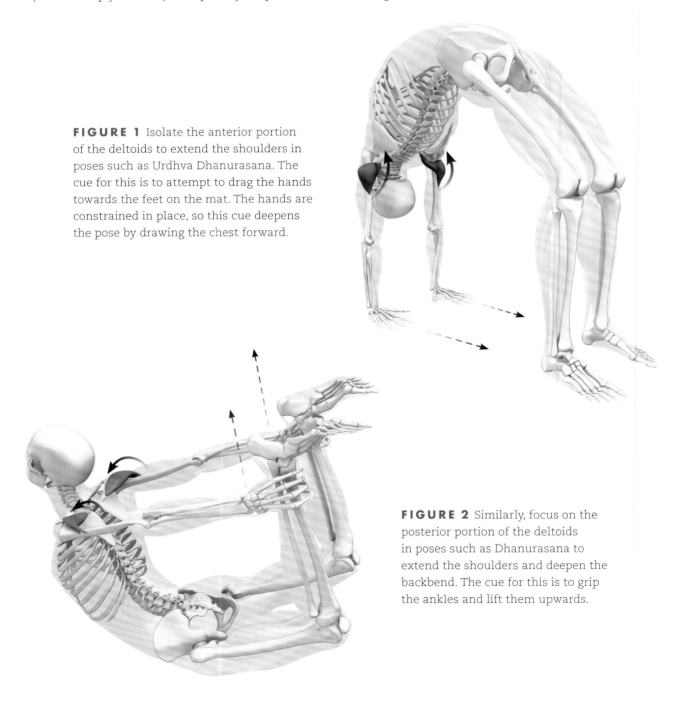

FIGURE 1 Isolate the anterior portion of the deltoids to extend the shoulders in poses such as Urdhva Dhanurasana. The cue for this is to attempt to drag the hands towards the feet on the mat. The hands are constrained in place, so this cue deepens the pose by drawing the chest forward.

FIGURE 2 Similarly, focus on the posterior portion of the deltoids in poses such as Dhanurasana to extend the shoulders and deepen the backbend. The cue for this is to grip the ankles and lift them upwards.

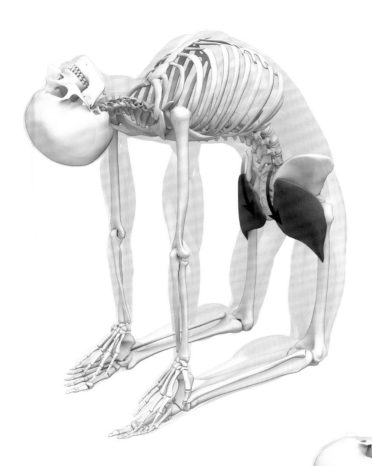

FIGURE 3 Use the prime mover muscles to position the major joints in yoga poses. For example, the hips extend in backbends. The gluteus maximus is the prime mover for extending the hip. Engage this muscle by tucking the tailbone and contracting the buttocks. This not only efficiently positions the hips, but also tilts the sacrum downward (retroversion), thereby protecting against hyperextension of the lumbar spine. Furthermore, contracting the gluteals also produces reciprocal inhibition of the hip flexors, relaxing them into the stretch.

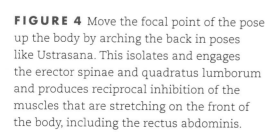

FIGURE 4 Move the focal point of the pose up the body by arching the back in poses like Ustrasana. This isolates and engages the erector spinae and quadratus lumborum and produces reciprocal inhibition of the muscles that are stretching on the front of the body, including the rectus abdominis.

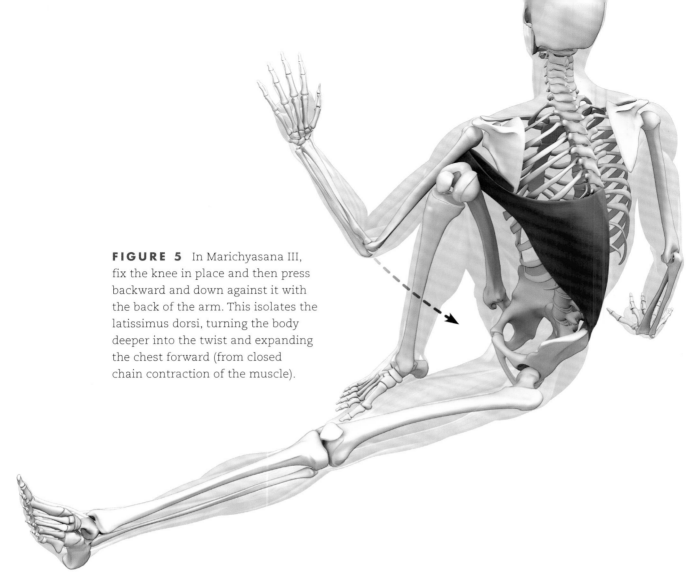

FIGURE 5 In Marichyasana III, fix the knee in place and then press backward and down against it with the back of the arm. This isolates the latissimus dorsi, turning the body deeper into the twist and expanding the chest forward (from closed chain contraction of the muscle).

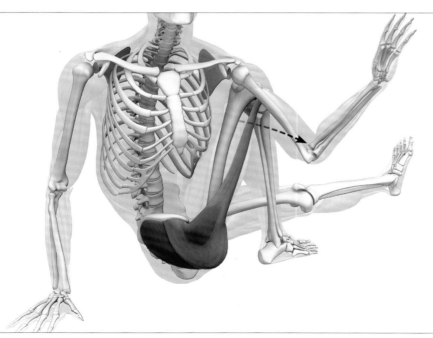

FIGURE 6 Fix the arm in place and then press the outside of the knee against it. This engages the tensor fascia lata and gluteus medius muscles—abductors of the hip. The fixed arm prevents the knee from moving outward (abducting), so the force of this contraction internally rotates the hip—a secondary action of the abductors. This turns the lower body away from the upper and deepens the twist.

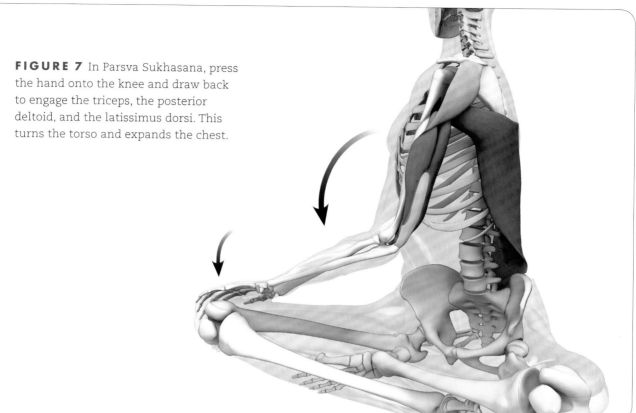

FIGURE 7 In Parsva Sukhasana, press the hand onto the knee and draw back to engage the triceps, the posterior deltoid, and the latissimus dorsi. This turns the torso and expands the chest.

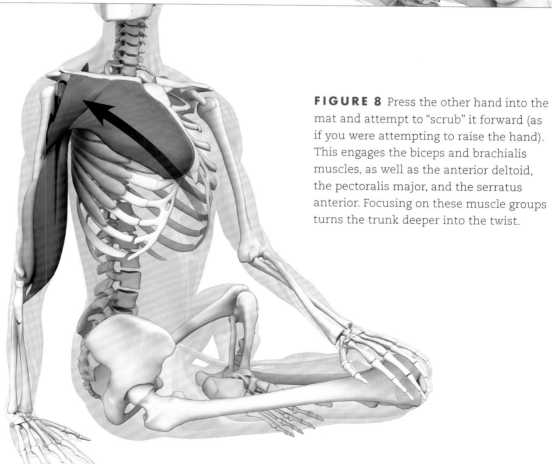

FIGURE 8 Press the other hand into the mat and attempt to "scrub" it forward (as if you were attempting to raise the hand). This engages the biceps and brachialis muscles, as well as the anterior deltoid, the pectoralis major, and the serratus anterior. Focusing on these muscle groups turns the trunk deeper into the twist.

KEY CONCEPT
THE MUSCLE SPINDLE

Knowledge of stretch receptors and spinal cord reflex arcs is an essential resource for yoga practitioners and teachers. These complex feedback mechanisms have three main components: a receptor at the muscular level that senses changes in tension and/or length, a sensory nerve to the spinal cord that relays this information to the central nervous system, and a motor nerve that conveys instructions to the muscle to relax or contract.

FIGURE 1 The muscle spindle is the sensory receptor in one such reflex arc. It detects changes in length and tension that take place within the muscle. For example, when you stretch a muscle in a yoga pose, its length and tension increase. The muscle spindle senses these changes and relays a message to the central nervous system. This message passes through the spinal cord and into an afferent nerve back to the muscle. The signal from this nerve is excitatory, causing contraction. The contraction prevents the muscle from lengthening further and protects against tearing.

This reflex arc is an unconscious physiological phenomenon that is triggered by a biomechanical event—stretching. Some of the muscle tension that you feel when you go into a stretch is due to this reflex. The muscle spindle reflex arc tapers off if you hold a stretch for a minute or so. It also diminishes if you contract its antagonist muscle. You can accelerate the acclimatization of the muscle spindle by backing off slightly from a deep stretch for three or four breaths. The muscle spindle will decrease its firing just as if you had held the stretch for a minute. You can then engage the antagonist muscles to go deeper into the pose.

FIGURE 1 Spinal Cord Reflex Arc

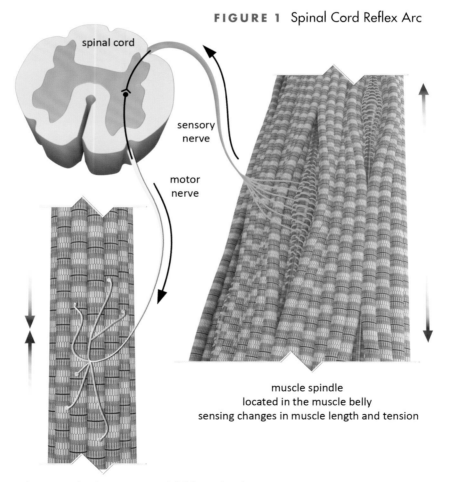

spinal cord

sensory nerve

motor nerve

muscle spindle
located in the muscle belly
sensing changes in muscle length and tension

muscle contracting in response to inhibitory signal

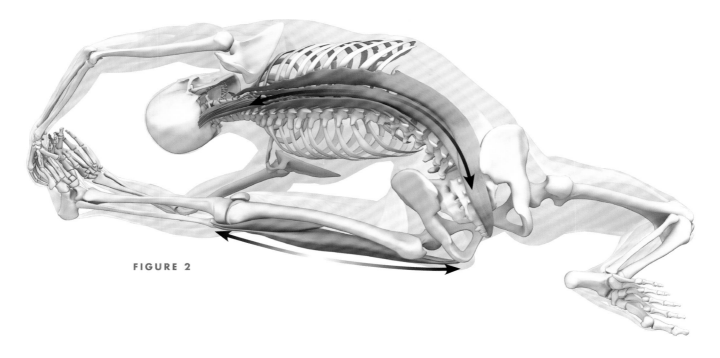

FIGURE 2

I illustrate this concept with Parighasana I. **FIGURE 2** shows the initial stretch of the hamstrings and erector spinae. **FIGURE 3** demonstrates backing out of the stretch slightly by bending the knee and releasing the hamstrings. **FIGURE 4** presents the final step of deepening the pose after the muscle spindles decrease their firing.

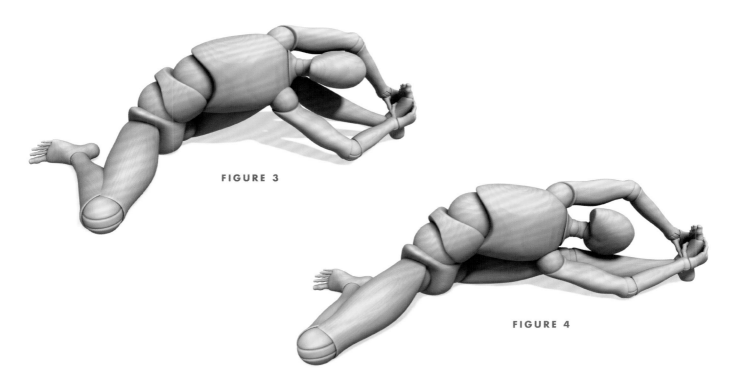

FIGURE 3

FIGURE 4

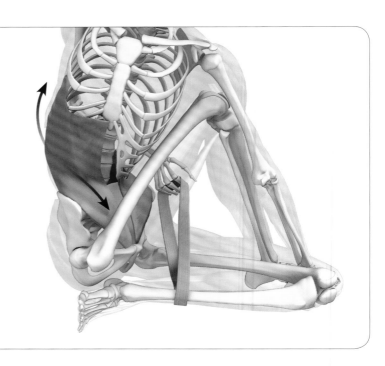

FIGURE 5 You can use this technique in Ardha Matsyendrasana and other twisting postures. Connecting the arms and legs produces a focal point in the trunk, stretching the abdominal obliques. This stimulates the muscle spindle stretch receptor, resulting in reflex contraction of these same muscles.

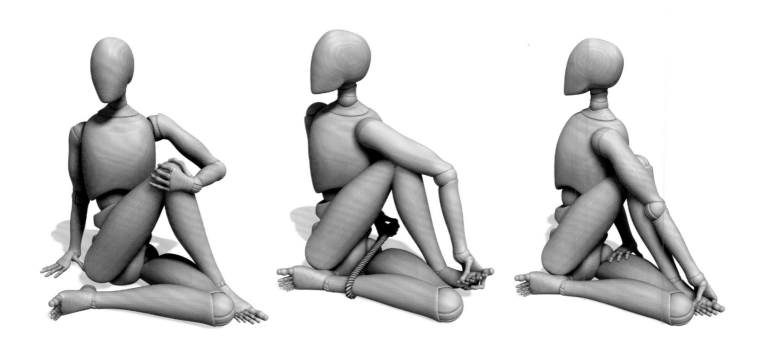

FIGURE 6 Partially back out of the pose while maintaining some stretch. This allows the muscle spindles to acclimate. Hold this position for several breaths, and then use the connection between the arms and legs to create a biomechanical lever point to deepen the asana.

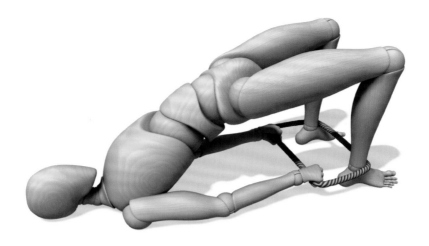

The hip flexors are a focal point for stretching in backbends. Acclimate the muscle spindles in this group by holding a shallower backbend such as Setu Bandha Sarvangasana (above) for several breaths before going into a deeper backbend, such as Urdhva Dhanurasana (below).

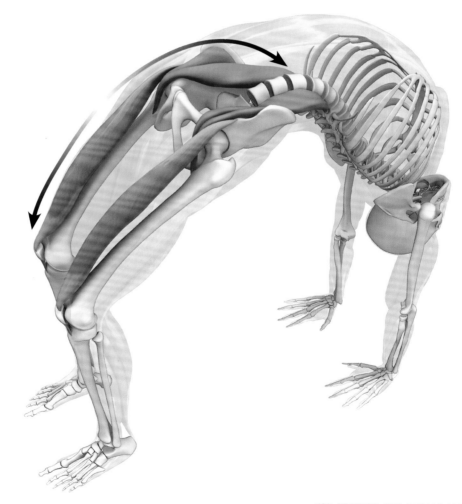

KEY CONCEPT
FACILITATED STRETCHES

Facilitated stretching works with another spinal cord reflex arc—the Golgi tendon organ. This sensory receptor is located at the muscle-tendon junction. The Golgi tendon organ detects increases in tension in the region and relays this information to the spinal cord, which then inhibits the muscle from contracting. This phenomenon, which protects the tendon from tearing, is known as the relaxation response. It can be used to create length in a muscle that you wish to stretch (**FIGURE 1**).

In facilitated stretching, we intentionally contract the muscle we are stretching. This increases firing of the Golgi tendon organ and augments the relaxation response. The response peaks at about two to three seconds after we stop contracting the target muscle, during which time we can take advantage of the "slack" that has been created and lengthen the muscle.

The technique works as follows:

1. Locate the muscle you want to lengthen.

2. Use biomechanics to stretch this muscle.

3. Maintain this stretch while contracting the target muscle for several smooth, deep breaths.

4. Release the contraction and then carefully take up the slack to deepen the pose.

FIGURE 1 Spinal Cord Reflex Arc

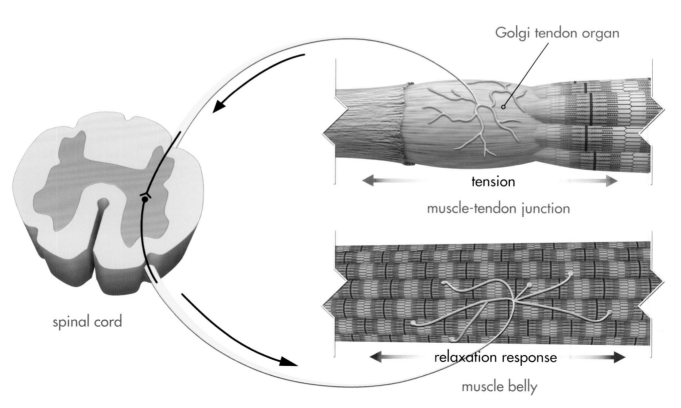

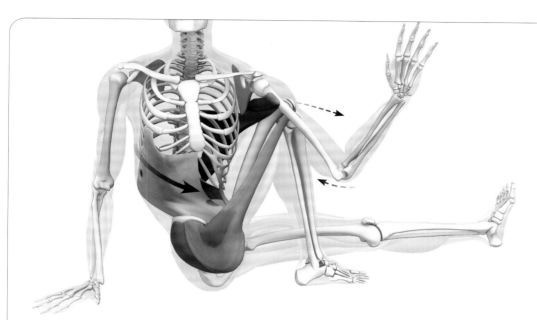

FIGURE 2 Marichyasana III stretches the oblique abdominals. You can use facilitated stretching to lengthen these muscles and deepen your twist. Do this by first going into the stretch to take the abdominal obliques out to length. Then contract the tensor fascia lata, gluteus medius, and latissimus dorsi by pressing the back of the arm into the knee. Hold this position and attempt to come out of the twist by engaging the abdominals.

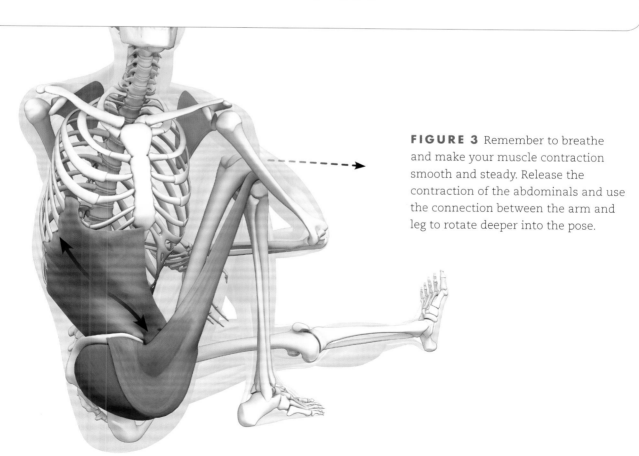

FIGURE 3 Remember to breathe and make your muscle contraction smooth and steady. Release the contraction of the abdominals and use the connection between the arm and leg to rotate deeper into the pose.

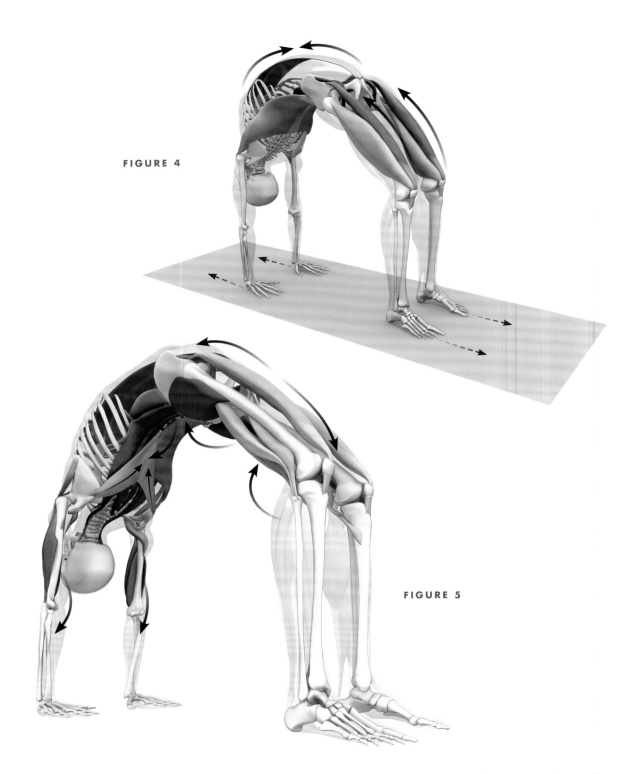

FIGURE 4

FIGURE 5

Backbends such as Urdhva Dhanurasana stretch the rectus abdominis, psoas, and rectus femoris muscles on the anterior trunk and pelvis. Facilitated stretching offers a method for lengthening these muscles. To apply this technique, attempt to scrub the hands away from the feet while at the same time engaging the abdominals (**FIGURE 4**). Maintain this action for a few steady breaths, and then deepen the pose by contracting the erector spinae, gluteus maximus, and hamstrings (**FIGURE 5**). Engaging these muscles augments the relaxation response with reciprocal inhibition of the stretching muscles identified above. This is an example of sequentially combining spinal cord reflexes to deepen a yoga pose.

KEY CONCEPT
KEY CO-ACTIVATIONS

Co-activation is the process in which we engage two or more muscles simultaneously. These can be an agonist/antagonist muscle group on either side of a joint or can be muscles separated at a distance. The effect of co-activation can both deepen and stabilize a pose.

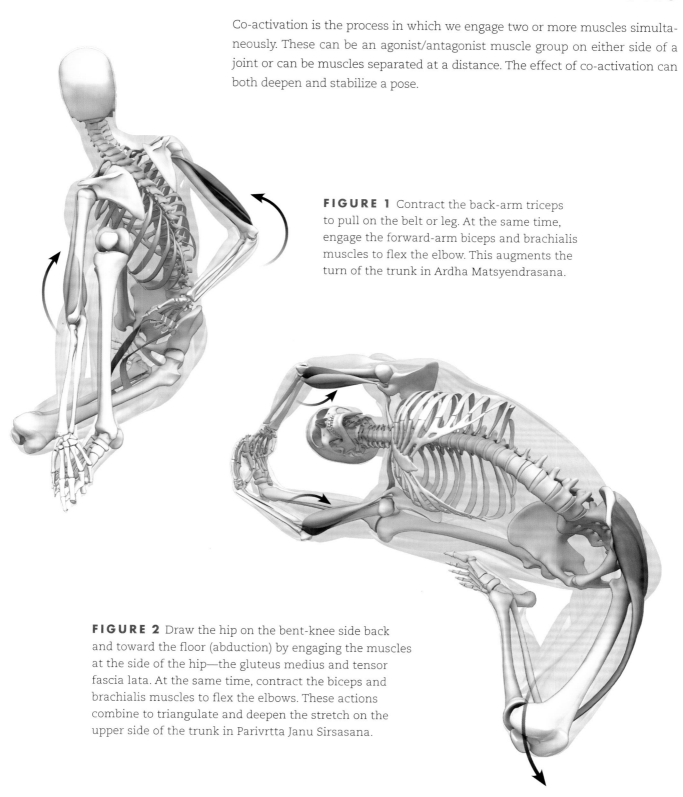

FIGURE 1 Contract the back-arm triceps to pull on the belt or leg. At the same time, engage the forward-arm biceps and brachialis muscles to flex the elbow. This augments the turn of the trunk in Ardha Matsyendrasana.

FIGURE 2 Draw the hip on the bent-knee side back and toward the floor (abduction) by engaging the muscles at the side of the hip—the gluteus medius and tensor fascia lata. At the same time, contract the biceps and brachialis muscles to flex the elbows. These actions combine to triangulate and deepen the stretch on the upper side of the trunk in Parivrtta Janu Sirsasana.

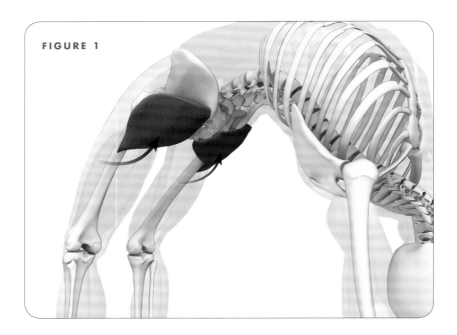

FIGURE 1

The form of any backbend includes extension of the hip joint. Thus it is useful to contract the gluteus maximus in these poses (**FIGURE 1**). This efficiently extends the hips, tilts the pelvis down, and produces reciprocal inhibition of the hip flexors—one of the muscle groups stretching in this pose category.

The disadvantage of contracting the gluteus maximus in backbends is that it also externally rotates the hip. Contracting it can cause the knees to splay apart, an undesirable effect in the pose. You can sequentially co-activate muscles to counteract this splaying, while retaining the benefits of engaging the gluteus maximus in backbends (**FIGURES 2 AND 3**).

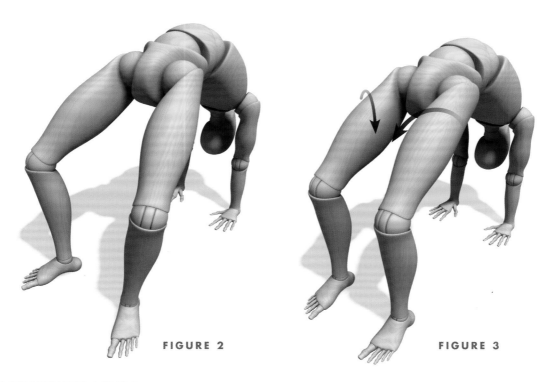

FIGURE 2   FIGURE 3

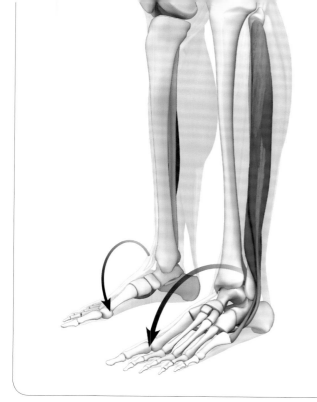

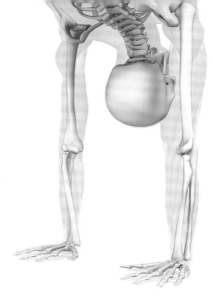

FIGURE 4 Begin by pressing the balls of the feet into the mat. This cue engages the peroneus longus and brevis muscles at the sides of the lower legs and fixes the feet in place.

▼ **FIGURE 5** Next, attempt to drag the feet apart (abduction). The feet won't move because they are fixed on the mat, but this action engages the tensor fascia lata and gluteus medius muscles. In addition to being hip abductors, these muscles also internally rotate the hip. This cue is critical to counteracting the external rotation moment created by the gluteus maximus. Attempting to abduct the hips also internally rotates them.

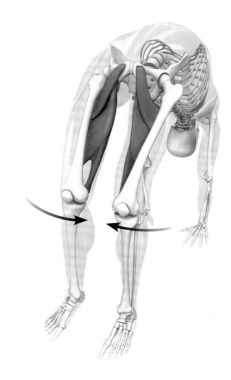

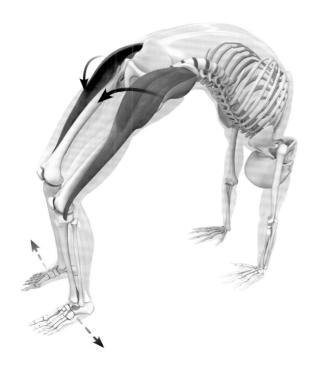

▲ **FIGURE 6** Finally, draw the knees towards one another by engaging the adductors on the inner thighs. Remember that the adductors synergize the gluteus maximus in externally rotating the hips and can contribute to splaying the knees. This is why it's essential to co-activate the tensor fascia lata and gluteus medius, as described in **FIGURE 5**.

KEY CONCEPT
BANDHAS

You can co-activate muscle groups to produce bandhas or "locks" throughout the body. These locks become focal points in the pose, both mentally and physically. In addition, bandhas stabilize the joints and stimulate the sensory nerves, accentuating the imprint of the pose on the brain. Facilitated stretching and co-activation are closely related—both can be used to create bandhas.

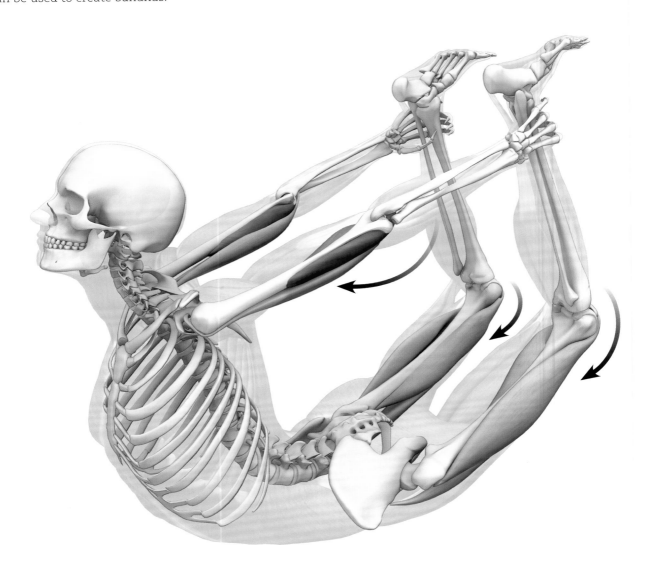

FIGURE 1 illustrates using co-activation in Dhanurasana. Contract the biceps and brachialis muscles to flex the elbows while engaging the quadriceps to straighten the knees. These actions stabilize and deepen the pose.

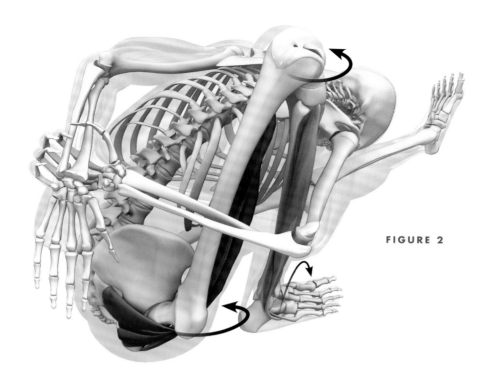

FIGURE 2

Simultaneously turn the trunk in one direction and rotate the pelvis and lower extremities in the other in Marichyasana I. This produces a bandha that is felt as a "wringing" effect across the torso. Experience this by pressing the ball of the bent-leg foot into the mat to engage the peroneus longus and brevis muscles. Then squeeze the lower leg against the thigh using the outside hamstrings (the biceps femoris). Next, externally rotate the hip by tucking the tailbone to engage the deep external hip rotators. These co-activations combine to externally rotate the bent leg at the hip (**FIGURE 2**). Hold this position and engage the abdomen to turn the trunk in the other direction (**FIGURE 3**). Feel how these actions produce a bandha across the abdomen and pelvis.

FIGURE 3

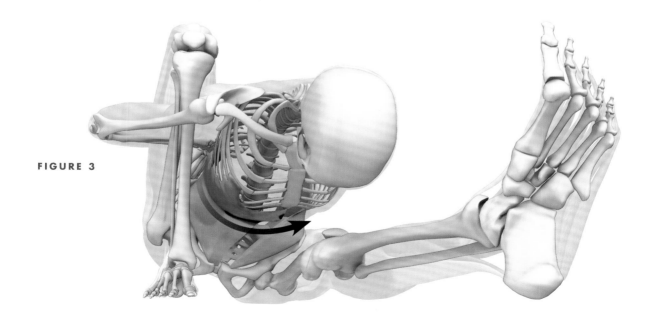

Use bandhas and co-activation to protect the lumbar spine and generate stability during backbends. Once you are in a pose like Ustrasana, gently engage the abdominal muscles (**FIGURE 1**). This has several beneficial effects. First, it produces a facilitated stretch of the abdominals. Next, it compresses the abdominal organs against the lumbar spine, supporting and protecting it against hyperextension. This is known as the abdominal "air-bag" effect (**FIGURE 2**). Finally, engaging the rectus abdominis pulls on the pubic bone and tilts the pelvis back and down into retroversion. This action counters hyperextension of the lumbar spine.

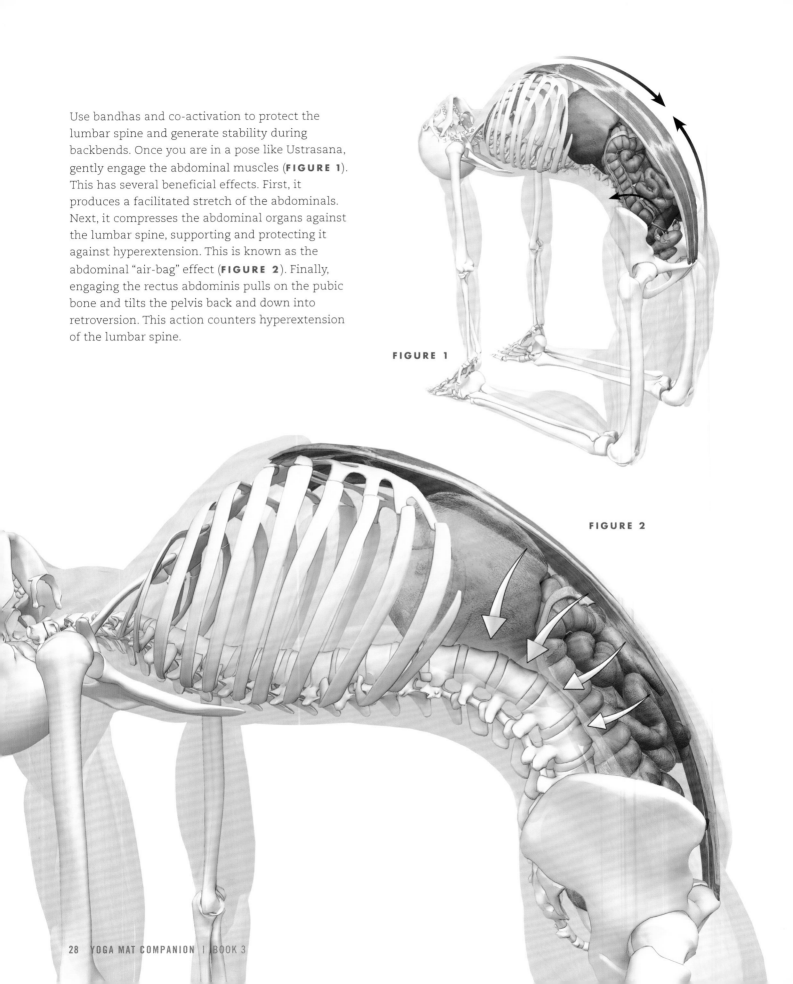

FIGURE 1

FIGURE 2

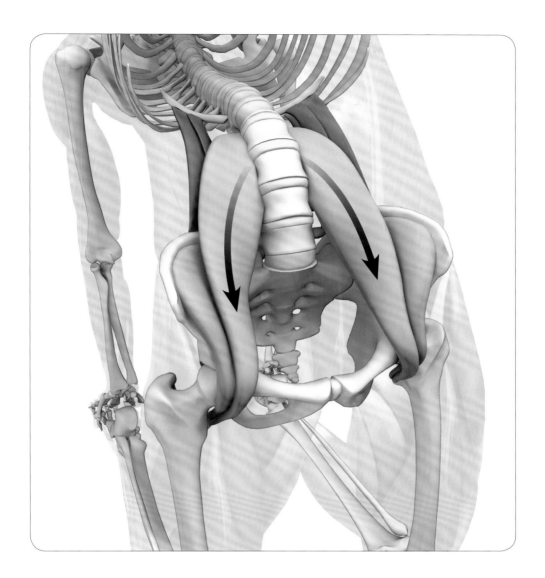

FIGURE 3 illustrates the relationship of the psoas and quadratus lumborum muscles to the lumbar spine. Arching the lower back contracts the quadratus lumborum. This muscle is neurologically connected to the psoas major, so that they automatically engage together to support the lumbar region. Take advantage of this relationship by attempting to slightly flex the hips once you are deep in a backbend. This action augments the contraction of the psoas major produced by arching the back.

THE
BANDHA YOGA
CODEX

EACH YOGA POSTURE HAS ITS OWN UNIQUE FORM AND FUNCTION. MUSCLES THAT engage in one posture may be stretching in another. For this reason it helps to have a road map for navigating your way to the optimal pose. Better still is the ability to create your own road map. The Bandha Yoga Codex shows you how to do this.

There are five elements to every asana. These are the joint positions, the muscles that engage to produce these positions, the muscles that stretch, the breath, and the bandhas. Understanding the joint positions enables you to determine the muscles that produce the posture. Engage the prime movers to sculpt the pose, and polish it with the synergists. Once you know the prime movers, you can identify the muscles that are stretching. Apply physiological techniques to lengthen these muscles and create mobility to deepen the pose.

Then there is the breath. In virtually every posture we can benefit from expanding the chest. Combine the accessory muscles of breathing with the action of the diaphragm to increase the volume of the thorax. This improves oxygenation of the blood and removes energetic blockages in the subtle body.

The bandhas are the finishing touch. Co-activate the muscle groups that produce the joint positions and you will create bandhas throughout the body. Then connect these peripheral locks to the core bandhas. This produces stability in the pose and accentuates the sensory imprint of the asana on the mind.

The Bandha Yoga Codex is a five-step process that teaches how to identify these elements and decode any pose. This is your guide to creating a road map for combining science and yoga. I use Dhanurasana to illustrate the Codex on the following pages.

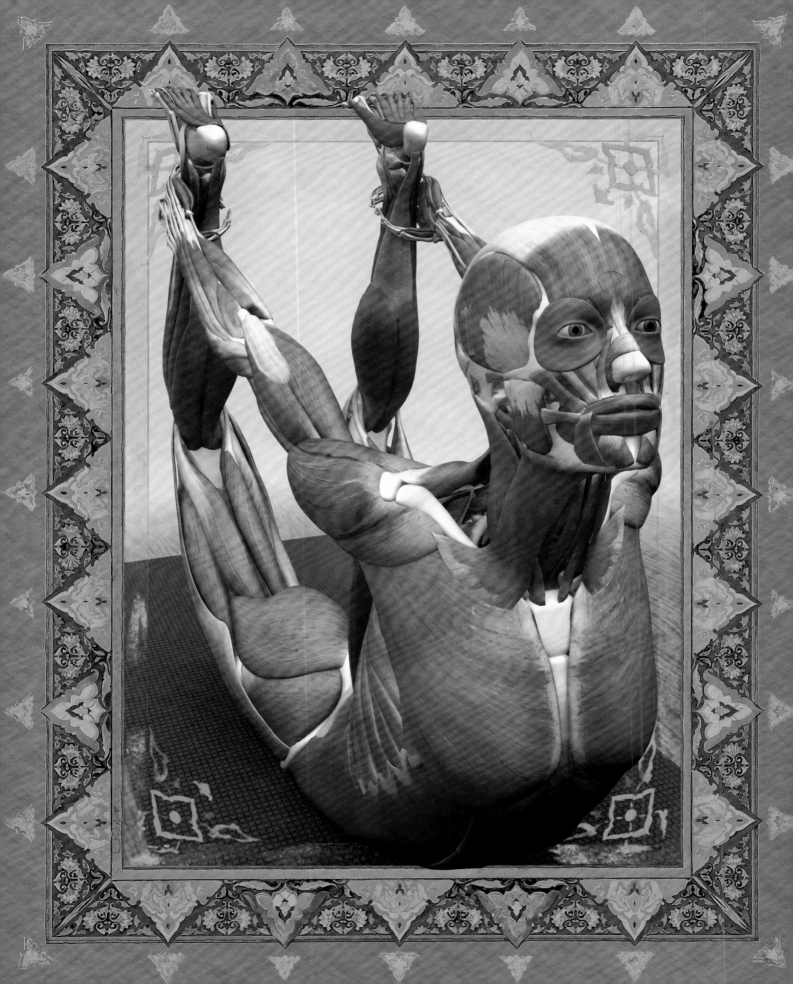

बन्ध योग

The Bandha Yoga Codex

— 1 —

Define the position of the joints in the pose.

— 2 —

Identify the prime mover muscles that act
on the joints to create the pose.
Contract these muscles to align and
stabilize the skeleton.

— 3 —

Identify the antagonist muscles
of the prime movers.
Stretch these muscles to create flexibility.

— 4 —

Expand the chest.

— 5 —

Create a Bandha.

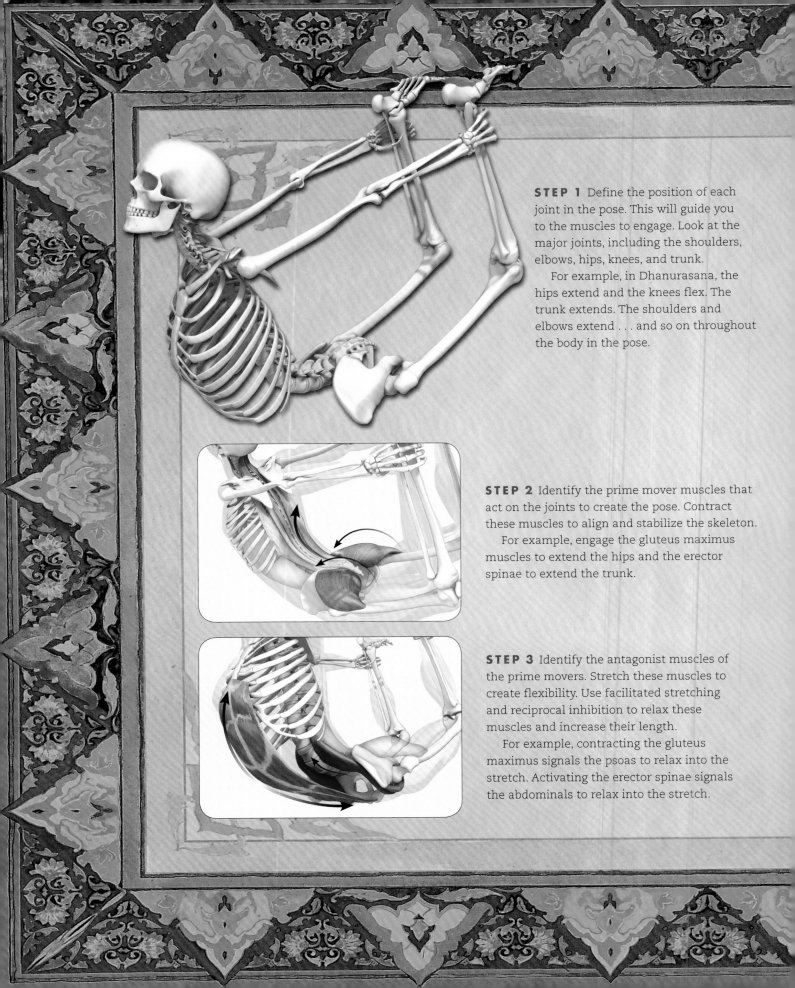

STEP 1 Define the position of each joint in the pose. This will guide you to the muscles to engage. Look at the major joints, including the shoulders, elbows, hips, knees, and trunk.

For example, in Dhanurasana, the hips extend and the knees flex. The trunk extends. The shoulders and elbows extend . . . and so on throughout the body in the pose.

STEP 2 Identify the prime mover muscles that act on the joints to create the pose. Contract these muscles to align and stabilize the skeleton.

For example, engage the gluteus maximus muscles to extend the hips and the erector spinae to extend the trunk.

STEP 3 Identify the antagonist muscles of the prime movers. Stretch these muscles to create flexibility. Use facilitated stretching and reciprocal inhibition to relax these muscles and increase their length.

For example, contracting the gluteus maximus signals the psoas to relax into the stretch. Activating the erector spinae signals the abdominals to relax into the stretch.

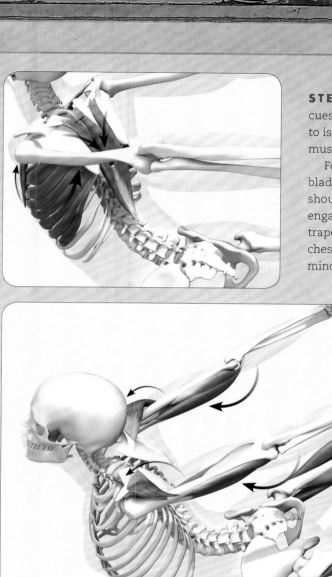

STEP 4 Expand the chest. Use the cues in this book to train yourself to isolate and engage the accessory muscles of breathing.

For example, draw the shoulder blades toward the midline and the shoulders away from the ears by engaging the rhomboids and lower trapezius. Then lift and expand the chest by contracting the pectoralis minor and serratus anterior muscles.

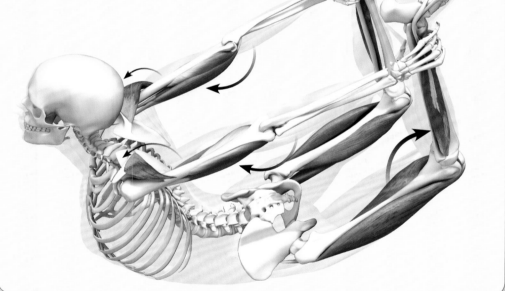

STEP 5 Create a bandha. This "locks" or stabilizes the pose, strengthens the muscles, and stimulates the nervous system.

For example, engage the peroneus longus and brevis muscles to evert the feet and lock the grip on the ankles. Then activate the quadriceps to attempt to extend the knees. At the same time, contract the posterior deltoids to lift the arms and the biceps and brachialis muscles to flex the elbows. Hold these actions for a breath or two. Feel how they deepen trunk extension and stabilize Dhanurasana.

BACKBENDS

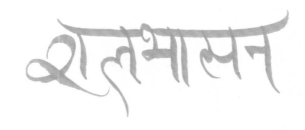

SALABHASANA

LOCUST POSE

AT FIRST GLANCE, SALABHASANA APPEARS TO BE AN EASY POSE. NEVERTHELESS, it requires significant flexibility and muscular effort to perform. Coupled joint rhythm is illustrated in Locust Pose, as the hips extend and the pelvis tilts back and down. At the same time, the lumbar spine also extends, countering the retroverted pelvis. Unlike backbends such as Ustrasana and Dhanurasana, there is no direct link between the upper and lower extremities that can be used to create leverage. In the version illustrated here, the backs of the hands press down on the floor, but they are at a mechanical disadvantage to generate much force to lift the chest. This is because the anterior deltoids—the muscles that raise the arms in front of the body—are in a lengthened state, such that cross-bridging on the molecular level is not optimal for strong contraction. Try anyway, as this builds strength and awareness in the muscles at the fronts of the shoulders.

The gluteals draw the pelvis back and down into retroversion, while at the same time lifting the femurs and extending the hips. The hamstrings synergize both actions by virtue of their origins on the ischial tuberosities and insertions on the lower legs. Squeeze the knees together to activate the adductor group. The most posterior of this group is the adductor magnus, which also synergizes the hamstrings and gluteus maximus to extend the femurs. Using the adductors to squeeze the knees together increases the force of contraction of other muscles, including the gluteus maximus and hamstrings—a phenomenon known as recruitment.

The weight of the body squeezes the abdomen, compressing its contents and raising intra-abdominal pressure. This creates a light resistance on the diaphragm from below, thus strengthening it. Once you are deeply in the asana, gently engage the rectus and transversus abdominis muscles to produce the abdominal "air bag" effect on the lumbar spine, protecting it and stabilizing the pose.

BASIC JOINT POSITIONS

- The elbows extend.
- The forearms pronate.
- The knees extend.
- The ankles plantar flex.

- The shoulders extend.
- The hips extend, internally rotate, and adduct.
- The trunk extends.

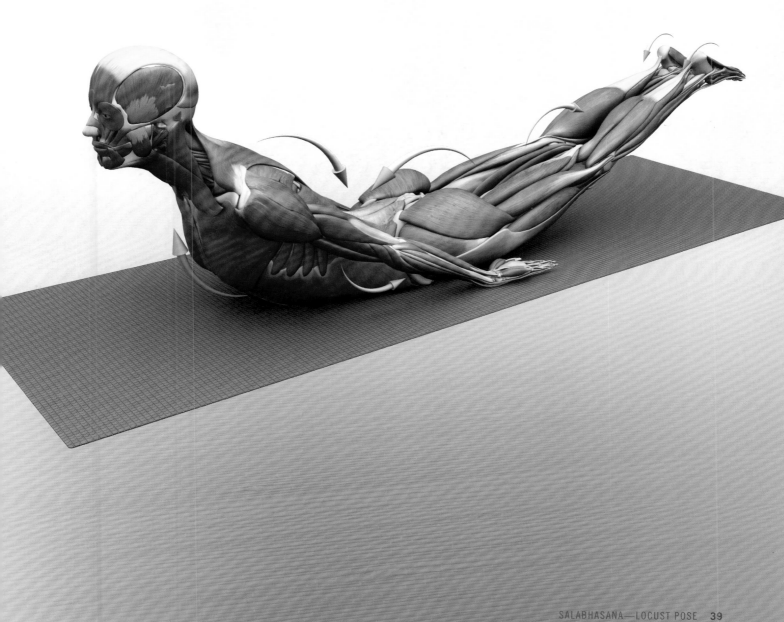

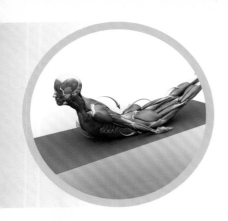

Salabhasana Preparation

Deconstruct the pose. First, lift the arms and chest while keeping the pelvis and thighs on the floor. Feel the muscles that engage in this variation. Then isolate the lower body by lifting the legs while keeping the arms and chest on the floor. Place the forearms on the mat and try to "scrub" back toward the pelvis with the elbows. Feel how this opens the chest. Lift the legs and squeeze them together. You can also place a bolster or blanket under the chest or thighs as you strengthen the muscles on the back to produce the force needed to create the final pose.

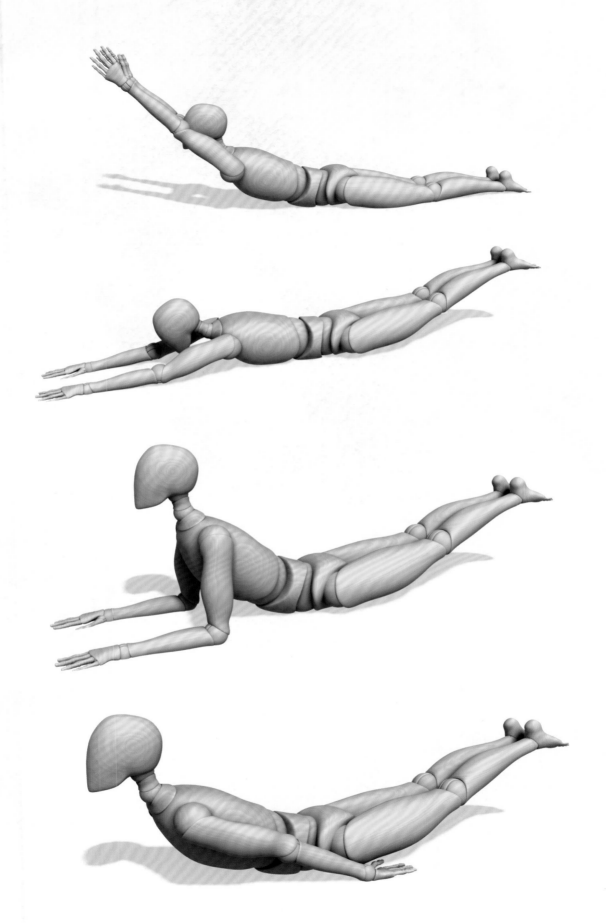

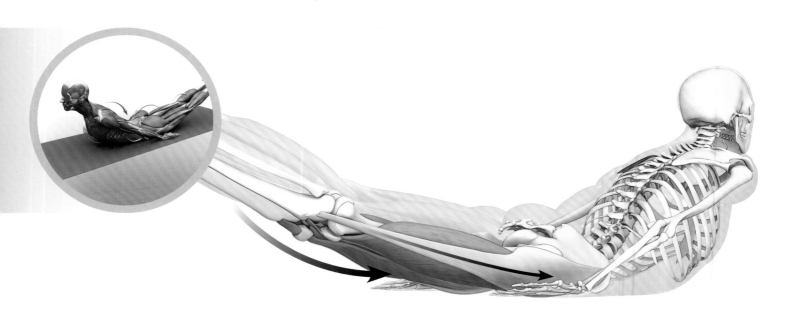

▲ **STEP 1** Activate the quadriceps to extend the knees. The tensor fascia lata synergizes this action. There is a tendency to turn the lower legs outward in this pose—as with all poses that use the gluteus maximus to extend the hips. This manifests in the kneecaps facing outward when ideally we want them to face a neutral direction. The tensor fascia lata counteracts this by internally rotating the femurs. A cue for isolating and contracting this muscle is to imagine pressing the outside edges of the feet into an immovable object, as if attempting to draw them away from the midline. This engages the abductor component of the tensor fascia lata and gluteus medius. Resist this by pressing the knees together, and note how the thighs roll inward, bringing the kneecaps more toward neutral.

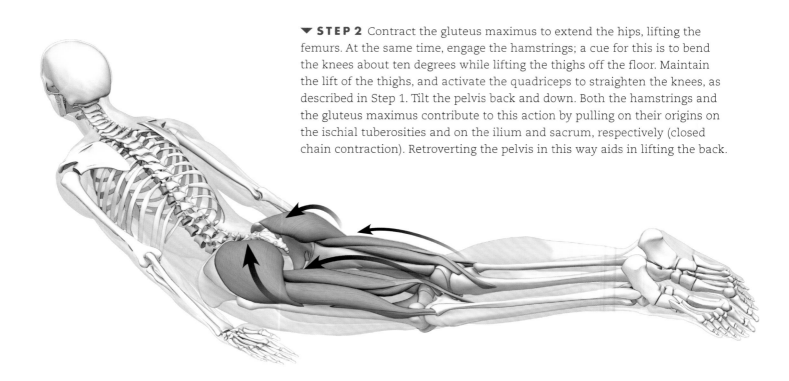

▼ **STEP 2** Contract the gluteus maximus to extend the hips, lifting the femurs. At the same time, engage the hamstrings; a cue for this is to bend the knees about ten degrees while lifting the thighs off the floor. Maintain the lift of the thighs, and activate the quadriceps to straighten the knees, as described in Step 1. Tilt the pelvis back and down. Both the hamstrings and the gluteus maximus contribute to this action by pulling on their origins on the ischial tuberosities and on the ilium and sacrum, respectively (closed chain contraction). Retroverting the pelvis in this way aids in lifting the back.

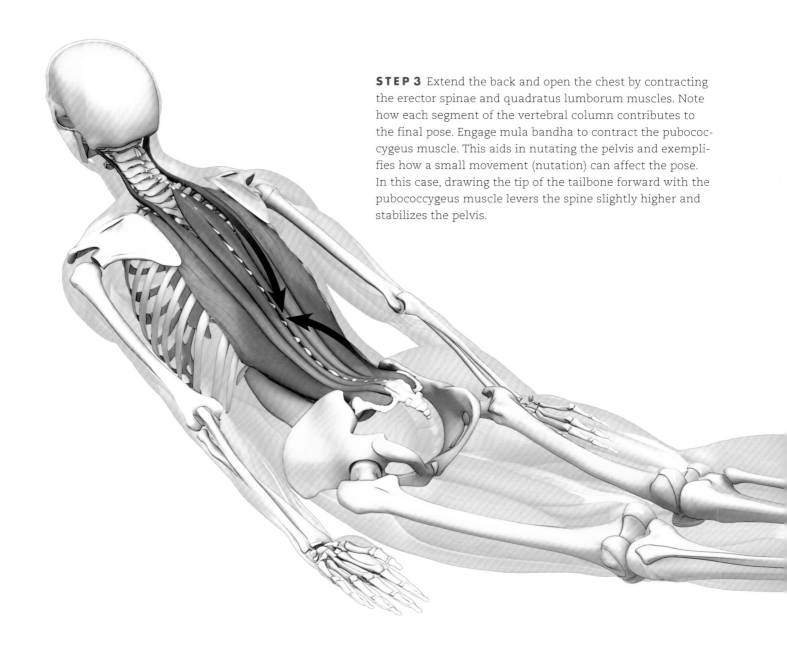

STEP 3 Extend the back and open the chest by contracting the erector spinae and quadratus lumborum muscles. Note how each segment of the vertebral column contributes to the final pose. Engage mula bandha to contract the pubococcygeus muscle. This aids in nutating the pelvis and exemplifies how a small movement (nutation) can affect the pose. In this case, drawing the tip of the tailbone forward with the pubococcygeus muscle levers the spine slightly higher and stabilizes the pelvis.

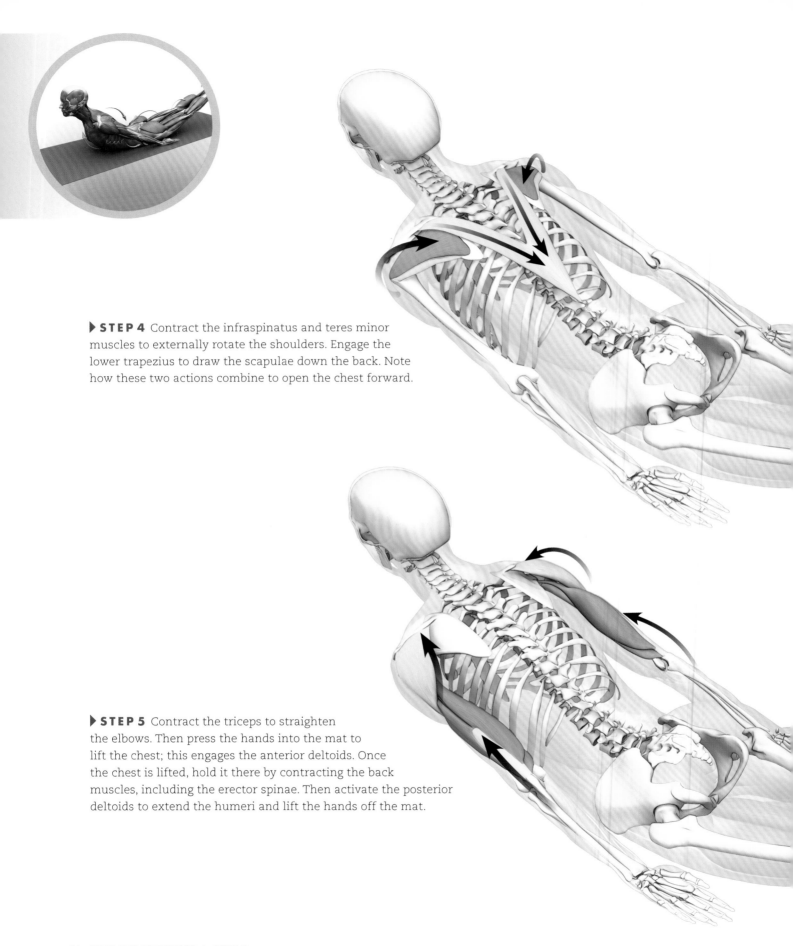

▶**STEP 4** Contract the infraspinatus and teres minor muscles to externally rotate the shoulders. Engage the lower trapezius to draw the scapulae down the back. Note how these two actions combine to open the chest forward.

▶**STEP 5** Contract the triceps to straighten the elbows. Then press the hands into the mat to lift the chest; this engages the anterior deltoids. Once the chest is lifted, hold it there by contracting the back muscles, including the erector spinae. Then activate the posterior deltoids to extend the humeri and lift the hands off the mat.

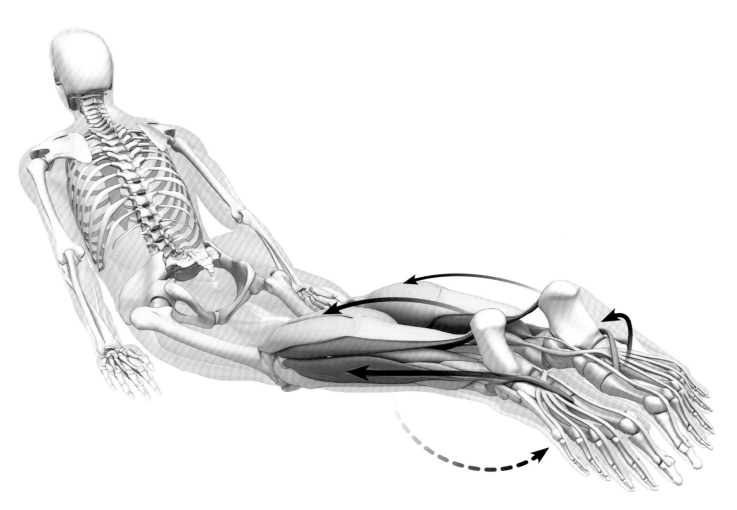

STEP 6 Flex the ankles to point the feet, so that the soles of the feet face upward. This activates the gastrocnemius/soleus complex. Slightly evert the ankles by contracting the peroneus longus and brevis muscles on the outer sides of the lower legs. Then counter this by engaging the tibialis posterior to create a slight inversion force. These actions combine to stabilize the ankles and open the soles of the feet, stimulating minor chakras located in this region.

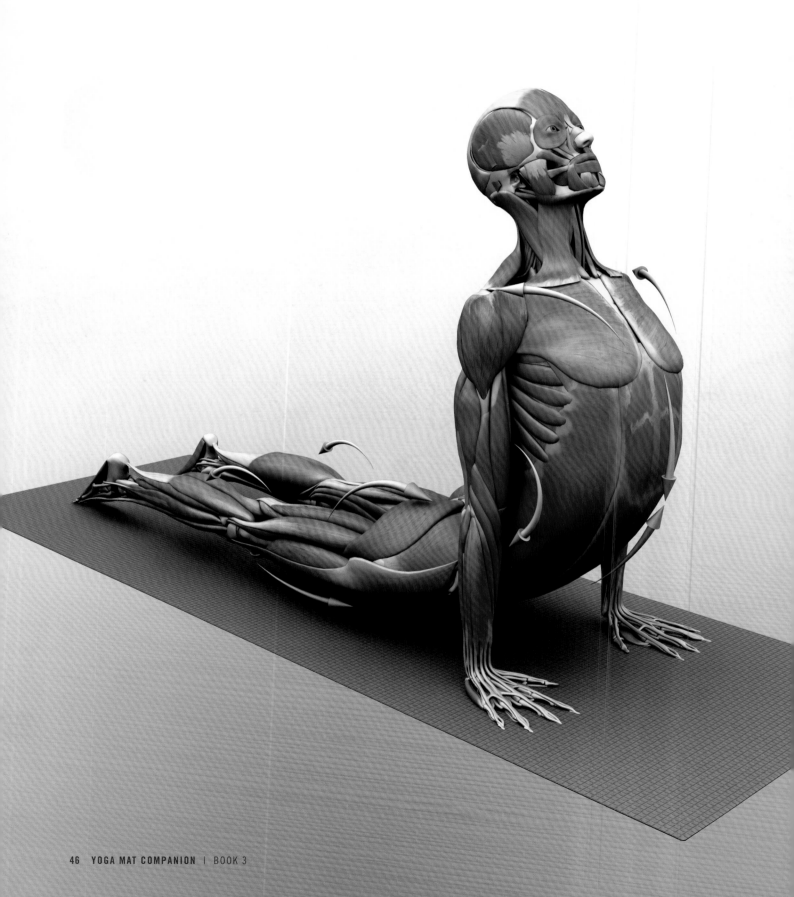

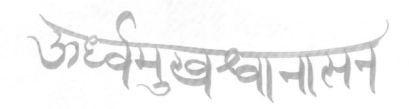

URDHVA MUKHA SVANASANA

UPWARD FACING DOG POSE

URDHVA MUKHA SVANASANA EXTENDS THE BACK OF THE BODY TO CREATE a focused stretch of the front. Each anatomical part contributes to the final pose. Concentrate on individual regions, and notice how each region affects distant parts. For example, feel how straightening the elbows extends the back and puts more pressure on the tops of the feet. Flex the feet and notice the affect on the front of the pelvis. Roll the shoulders back and observe the affect on the chest—how it opens and draws the pelvis forward. This is a good exercise in any pose, as it emphasizes how yoga works the entire body and not only one area.

BASIC JOINT POSITIONS

- The knees extend.
- The ankles plantar flex.
- The hips extend, internally rotate, and adduct.
- The elbows extend.
- The forearms pronate.
- The shoulders extend and externally rotate.
- The trunk extends.

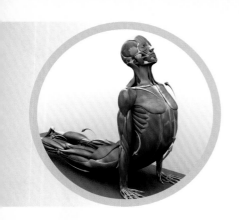

Urdhva Mukha Svanasana Preparation

At first, leave the thighs on the floor. Begin with the elbows bent and attempt to "scrub" backward on the mat toward the pelvis, drawing the chest forward. Roll the shoulders back and down. Begin to straighten the elbows by engaging the triceps. Press the mounds of the fingers (where the fingers meet the palms) into the mat to create a flexion moment at the wrists. These actions strengthen both the triceps and the muscles of the forearms. Lift and expand the chest forward.

Finally, straighten the arms and extend the knees to lift the pelvis off the mat. Attempt to scrub backward with the hands, just as you did with the elbows. This draws the chest forward from the lower and middle portions of the back.

Use the stretch illustrated here to lengthen the psoas and its synergists of hip flexion in preparation for Upward Facing Dog.

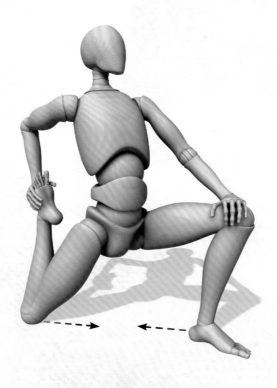

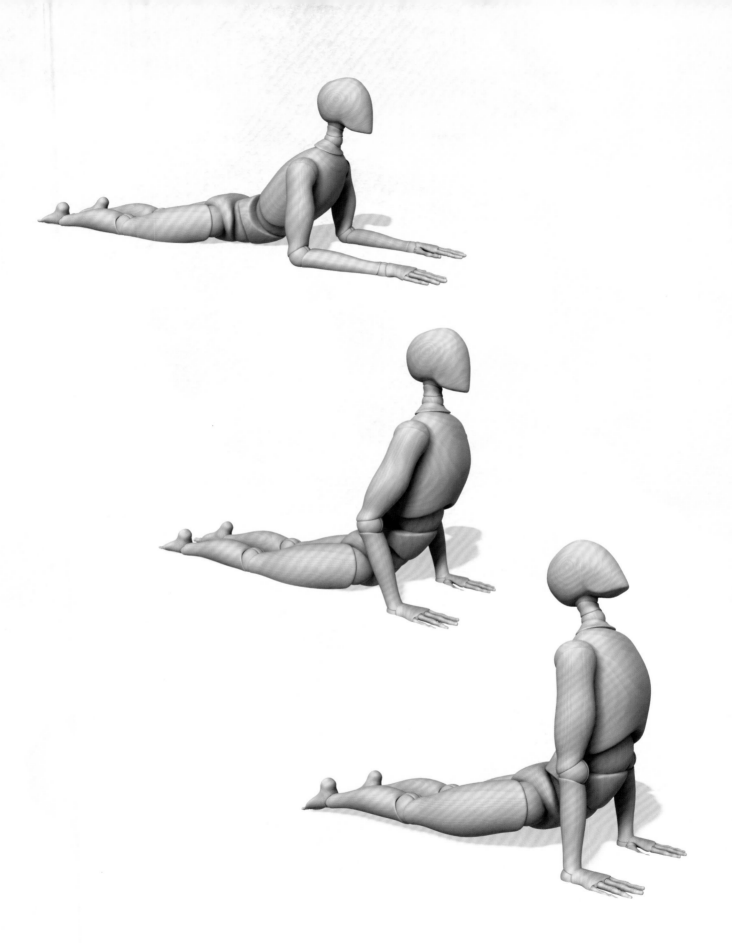

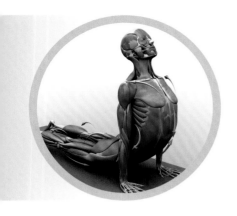

STEP 1 Engage the erector spinae to extend the vertebral column. Activate the gluteus maximus and medius to extend the hips and femurs. Engage mula bandha to contract the pubococcygeus and piriformis muscles and nutate the sacrum. This action aligns the sacrum and pelvis. The gluteus maximus will naturally turn the femurs outward. Step 2 illustrates how to counter this tendency by contracting the tensor fascia lata and anterior fibers of the gluteus medius. Attempt to draw the thighs together to activate the adductor magnus and synergize the gluteus maximus in extending the hips.

▶ **STEP 2** Activate the quadriceps to extend the knees. As with Locust Pose, this has the added benefit of anteverting the pelvis from the action of the rectus femoris. Engage the tensor fascia lata to synergize the quadriceps in extending the knees. The thighs tend to roll outward from the external rotational force of the gluteus maximus. Counteract this tendency by pressing the tops of the feet into the mat and attempting to drag them away from the midline. This engages fibers of the tensor fascia lata and gluteus medius that internally rotate the femurs, bringing the kneecaps to face downward.

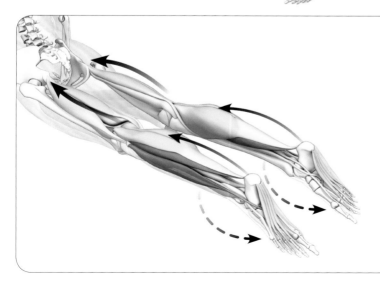

STEP 3 Contract the gastrocnemius/soleus complex to plantar flex the ankles. Counteract the tendency of the heels to roll outward by engaging the peroneus longus and brevis muscles at the sides of the lower legs to evert the feet. A cue for this is to activate the gluteus maximus and quadriceps while at the same time pressing the balls of the feet away from the pelvis. Stabilize the ankles by engaging the tibialis posterior muscles to balance this eversion with an inversion moment. Activate the hamstrings by attempting to lift the legs off the mat.

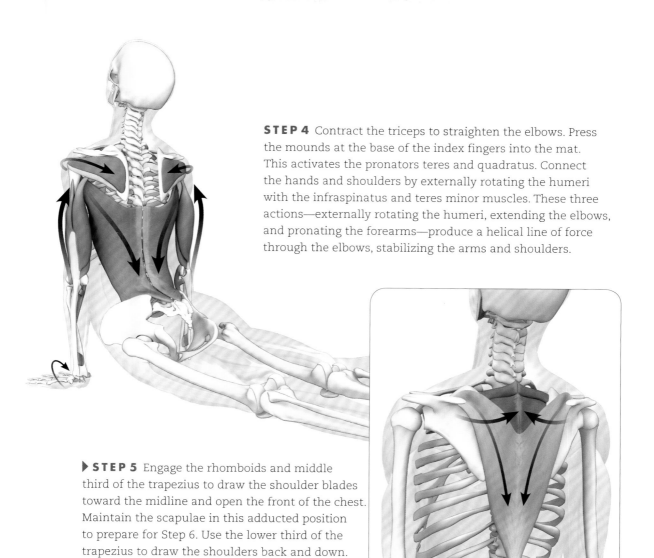

STEP 4 Contract the triceps to straighten the elbows. Press the mounds at the base of the index fingers into the mat. This activates the pronators teres and quadratus. Connect the hands and shoulders by externally rotating the humeri with the infraspinatus and teres minor muscles. These three actions—externally rotating the humeri, extending the elbows, and pronating the forearms—produce a helical line of force through the elbows, stabilizing the arms and shoulders.

▶ **STEP 5** Engage the rhomboids and middle third of the trapezius to draw the shoulder blades toward the midline and open the front of the chest. Maintain the scapulae in this adducted position to prepare for Step 6. Use the lower third of the trapezius to draw the shoulders back and down.

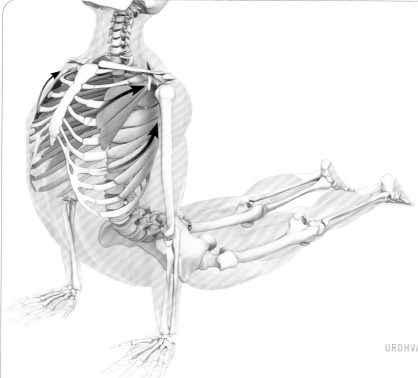

STEP 6 Finally, expand the ribcage by contracting the pectoralis minor and serratus anterior. In Step 5 we stabilized the shoulder blades with the rhomboids. Maintain this position and attempt to roll the shoulders forward while continuing to fix the scapulae toward the midline. Attempting to roll the shoulders forward while the scapulae are constrained produces closed chain contraction of the pectoralis minor. This draws the origin of the muscle on the ribcage upward, expanding the chest. Expand the chest outward from the sides to engage the serratus anterior. A cue for activating this muscle is to imagine pressing the arms outward against a door frame.

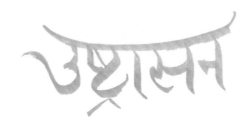

USTRASANA

CAMEL POSE

USTRASANA EXTENDS THE BACK OF THE BODY TO STRETCH THE FRONT. The shoulders draw back to link the hands to the soles of the feet, and the knees lever the body up and forward to deepen the pose. The thighs tend to drift backward in Ustrasana, decreasing the angle between the upper and lower legs. Contract the quadriceps to extend the knees. This brings the thighs perpendicular to the floor, deepening the backbend (especially when the hands are holding the bottoms of the feet). Review the section on facilitated stretches to see how isolated stretching of the fronts of the shoulders and hips can improve this pose.

Notice how the individual parts work together to deepen the asana. For example, combine the subplot of extending the shoulders with the subplot of extending the knees to "triangulate" the spinal extension. Then engage the abdominals to produce the abdominal "air bag" effect. This prevents hyper extension of the lumbar spine and aids to protect the lower back.

BASIC JOINT POSITIONS

- The knees flex.
- The ankles plantar flex.
- The hips extend, internally rotate, and adduct.
- The trunk extends.
- The shoulders extend.
- The elbows extend.
- The forearms supinate.

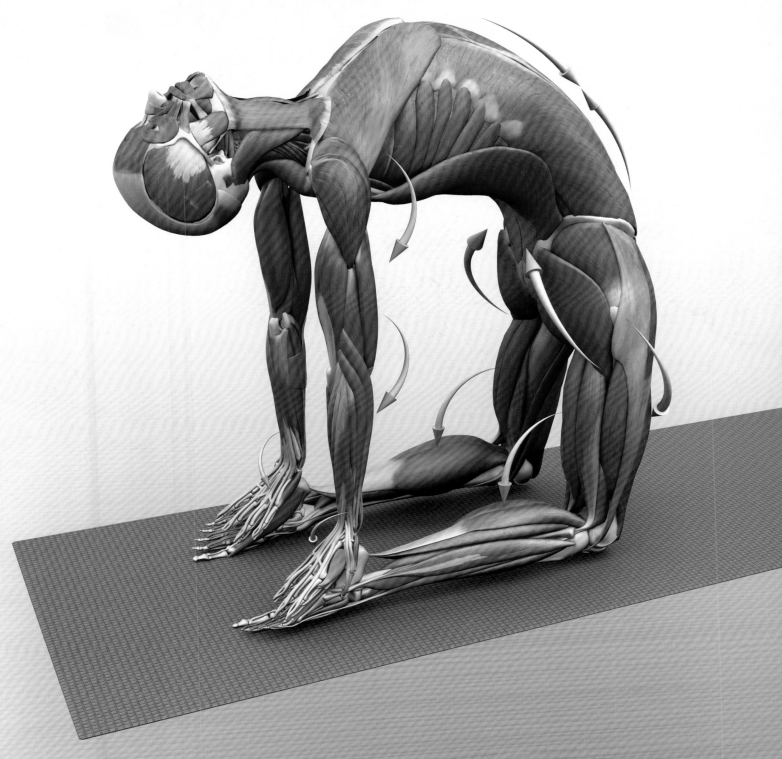

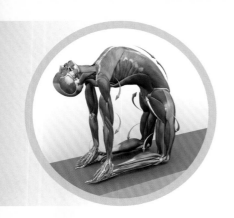

Ustrasana Preparation

Begin with the hands on the hips and draw the elbows back and towards each other. Press downward on the hips to lift the chest. Then begin to arch the spine. Because this is a fairly advanced pose, work in this intermediate position at first to condition the muscles that arch the back—the erector spinae and quadratus lumborum. Contract the quadriceps to extend the knees and bring the thighs to an upright position, perpendicular to the floor. Practice easing into and out of this position by pressing the shins down and attempting to straighten the knees. This levers the body upright.

Once you have a good sense of balance, let the arms fall back symmetrically toward the feet. If you're unable to reach the feet, then keep the hands on the hips. When you have gained sufficient flexibility, place the palms of the hands onto the soles of the feet. Take care not to rotate the body during this movement. Rotational movements while extending the spine, especially if unplanned, can result in injury. Maintain soft and steady breathing throughout.

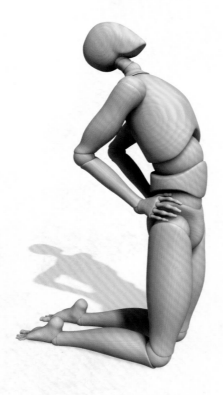

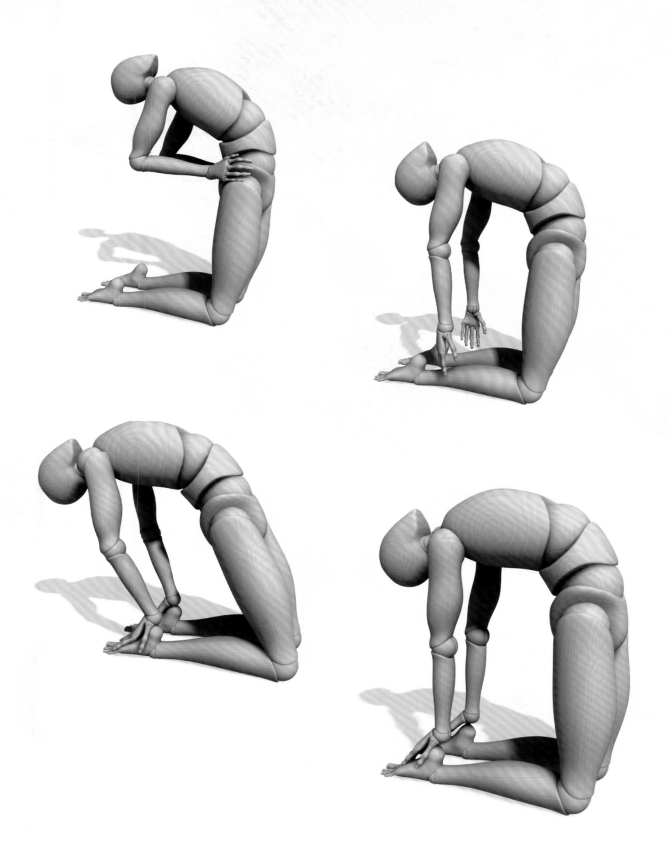

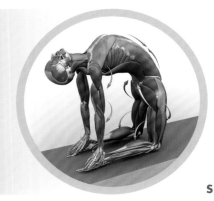

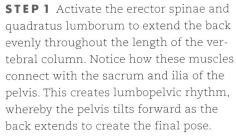

STEP 1 Activate the erector spinae and quadratus lumborum to extend the back evenly throughout the length of the vertebral column. Notice how these muscles connect with the sacrum and ilia of the pelvis. This creates lumbopelvic rhythm, whereby the pelvis tilts forward as the back extends to create the final pose.

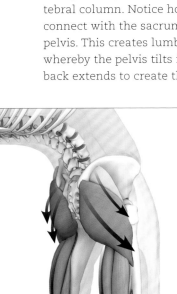

STEP 2 Engage the gluteus maximus to extend the hips and femurs. This also retroverts the pelvis, tilting it back and down and drawing it in an opposite direction to the back muscles described in Step 2. This combination of forces stabilizes the pelvis. The fibers of the posterior third of the gluteus medius assist the gluteus maximus in this movement. The posterior tilt of the pelvis helps to counteract hyperextension of the lumbar spine. The hamstrings synergize the actions of tilting the pelvis back and down and extending the femurs (when the lower legs are fixed on the mat). As you deepen the pose, relax the hamstrings, or they will bend the knees and draw the thighs away from their vertical position.

STEP 3 Engage the posterior deltoids to extend the shoulders. You can review this action in the muscle isolation section. Contract the infraspinatus and teres minor muscles to externally rotate the shoulders. Use the triceps to extend the elbows, and contract the supinator muscles of the forearms to rotate the palms so that the outer sides preferentially push down on the feet. Then balance the action of the supinators by pressing the mounds at the base of the index fingers into the soles, engaging the pronator teres and quadratus muscles of the forearms.

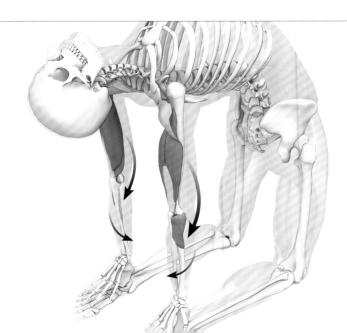

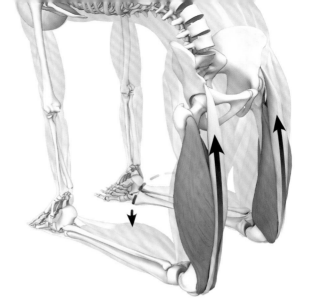

STEP 4 If the pelvis drifts backwards toward the lower legs, most people's instinct is to engage the buttocks to push it forward. This can actually draw the pelvis back more, because the gluteus maximus is tilting it back and down. A more efficient but less obvious action is to engage the quadriceps, as illustrated here. This increases the angle between the thighs and lower legs and easily levers the pelvis forward. The cue for engaging the quadriceps is to press the tops of the feet into the floor, as if trying to straighten the knees.

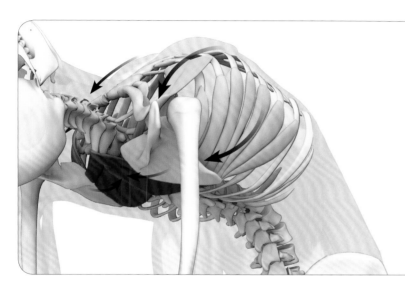

STEP 5 Contract the rhomboids to adduct the shoulder blades toward the midline, opening the chest upward. Then engage the pectoralis minor and serratus anterior to expand the ribcage. The cue for engaging the pectoralis minor is to constrain the scapulae backward in adduction against the spine, and then attempt to roll the shoulders forward. The shoulders will not move, so the force of the contraction is transmitted to the origin of the muscle on the ribcage, lifting it. To engage the serratus anterior, hold the scapulae in place and imagine pressing the hands outward against a door frame.

STEP 6 Finalize the pose by activating the rectus abdominis. This produces the abdominal "air bag" effect, wherein the increased intra-abdominal pressure supports the lumbar spine. The rectus abdominis also pulls upward on the pubic symphysis. This synergizes the action of the gluteus maximus in retroverting the pelvis, aiding to protect against lumbar hyperextension. Use the pubococcygeus and piriformis muscles to engage mula bandha and nutate the sacrum. This aligns the sacrum with the iliac bones, helping to prevent hyperextension of the lumbar spine.

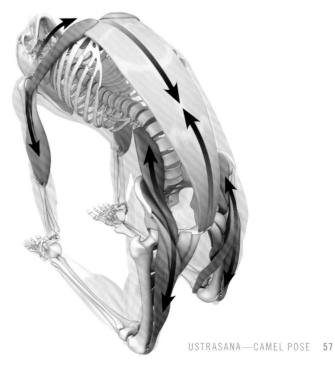

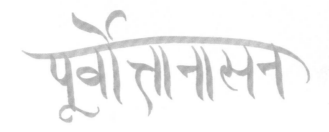

PURVOTTANASANA

INCLINED PLANE POSE

PURVOTTANASANA IS THE NEXT POSE IN THE PROGRESSIVE BACKBEND SERIES presented here. We started with Salabhasana and then worked our way into Urdhva Mukha Svanasana. Then we progressed to Dhanurasana and Ustrasana, both of which have the shoulders extended away from the back and the hands linked to the feet. Here the yoga mat connects the upper and lower extremities.

Purvottanasana combines upper body extension with a lift of the pelvis to lengthen the front of the body and strengthen the entire posterior kinetic chain. Straighten the elbows and extend the upper arms to open the chest. Press the soles of the feet into the floor and straighten the knees to form a bridge with the lower body; lift the pelvis toward the ceiling. Extend the femurs and hips and tuck the tail-bone back and down (retroversion) to open the front of the pelvis. Allow the neck to release and the head to drop back to relax the brain.

BASIC JOINT POSITIONS

- The shoulders extend and externally rotate.
- The elbows extend.
- The forearms pronate.
- The trunk and cervical spine extend.

- The hips extend, internally rotate, and adduct.
- The knees extend.
- The ankles plantar flex.

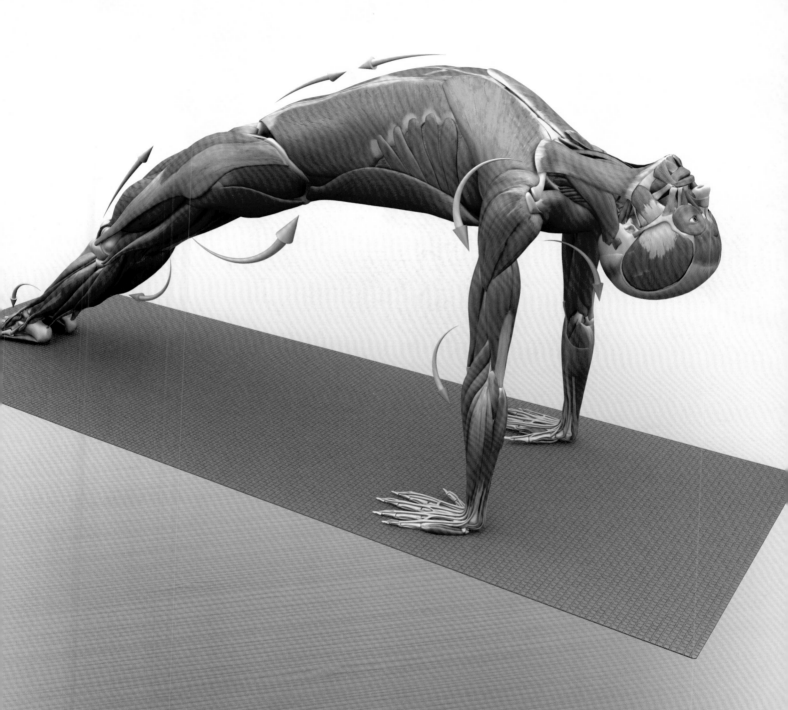

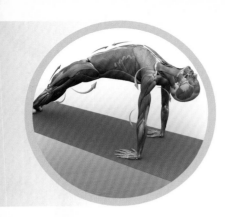

Purvottanasana Preparation

Purvottanasana stretches the flexor muscles at the fronts of the hips, including the psoas and its synergists. Isolate and lengthen these muscles to prepare for the pose using the facilitated stretch illustrated below.

Begin with the arms extending back from the body and the palms placed firmly on the mat. Be careful not to hyperextend the wrists. If you feel pain in the wrists, then bend the elbows slightly to take some of the extension out of the joints. Lift the chest. Then activate the buttocks and hamstring muscles to lift the pelvis. Keep the knees bent in this position, with the lower legs at right angles to the floor. Open the chest upwards and extend the elbows; let the head drop back. Work on this stage of the pose for as long as is necessary.

Finally, walk the feet out and straighten the knees. Flex the ankles to press the soles of the feet into the mat. Lift the buttocks and expand the chest. Ease out of the pose by bending the knees and elbows and carefully lowering to the floor.

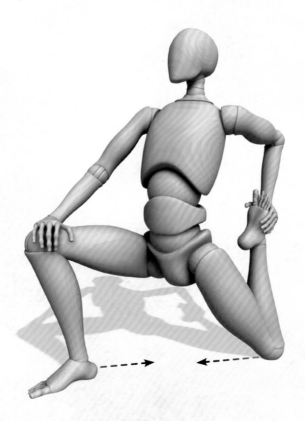

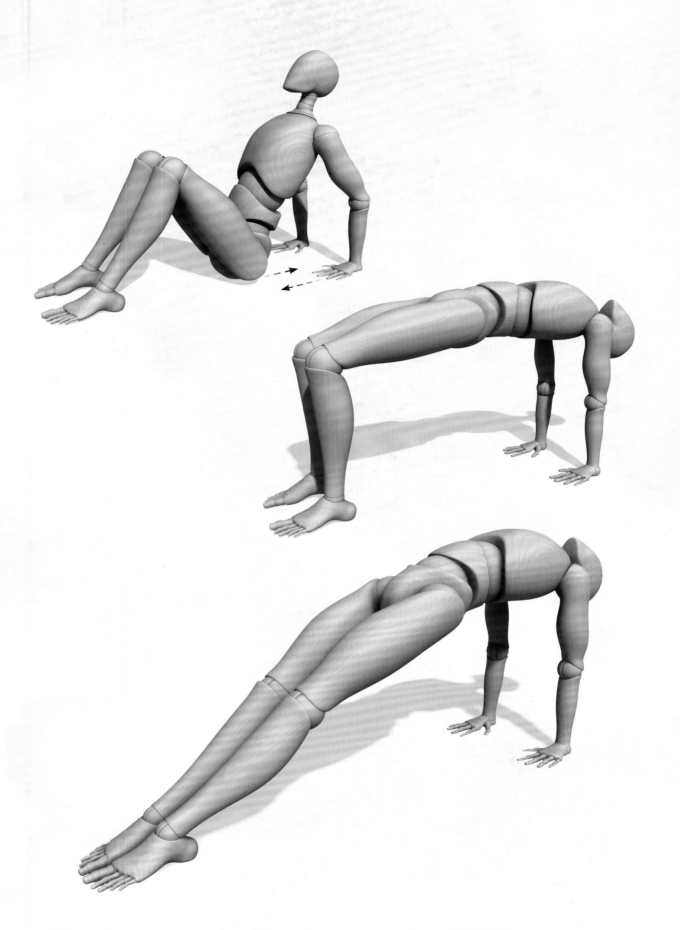

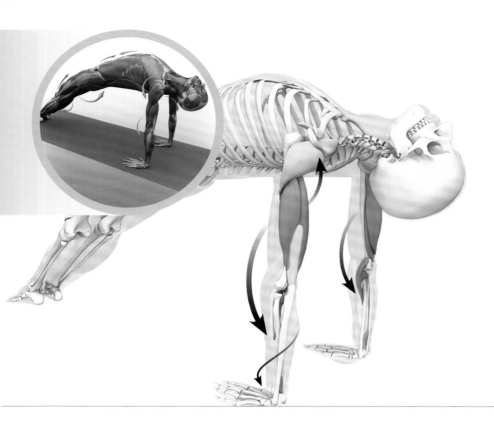

STEP 1 Pronate the forearms and flex the wrists to press the palms of the hands into the mat. Activate the pronators teres and quadratus to press the mounds at the base of the index fingers into the floor. Engage the triceps to straighten the elbows, and contract the posterior deltoids to extend the shoulders away from the back at the glenohumeral joint. Externally rotate the humeri by activating the infraspinatus and teres minor muscles. Because you have already internally rotated the forearms, this external rotation creates a stabilizing helical force from the shoulders, through the elbows, and into the palms of the hands.

STEP 2 Activate the gluteus maximus, medius, and minimus to extend the femurs and tilt the pelvis back and down into retroversion. Arch the back by contracting the erector spinae and quadratus lumborum muscles. Engaging the hamstrings aids in pressing the soles of the feet into the mat and causes an upward-directed force that synergizes the lift of the pelvis.

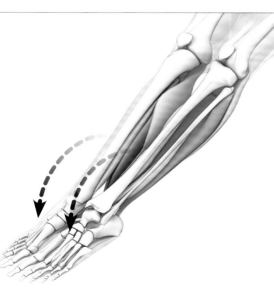

STEP 3 Activate the gastrocnemius and soleus muscles to plantar flex the ankles and press the feet into the floor. This requires some length in the antagonist muscles at the fronts of the lower legs that act to dorsiflex the ankles—the tibialis anterior and extensors hallucis and digitorum longus. Poses such as Virasana and Triang Mukhaikapada Paschimottanasana help to stretch these muscles. Press the balls of the feet into the mat by engaging the peroneus longus and brevis, which evert the ankles. Then spread the weight to the outer edges of the feet by contracting the tibialis posterior muscles. Creating both an eversion and inversion force at the ankles aids to stabilize the feet on the mat by spreading the weight across the soles.

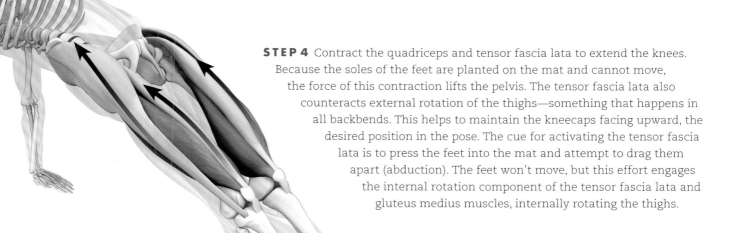

STEP 4 Contract the quadriceps and tensor fascia lata to extend the knees. Because the soles of the feet are planted on the mat and cannot move, the force of this contraction lifts the pelvis. The tensor fascia lata also counteracts external rotation of the thighs—something that happens in all backbends. This helps to maintain the kneecaps facing upward, the desired position in the pose. The cue for activating the tensor fascia lata is to press the feet into the mat and attempt to drag them apart (abduction). The feet won't move, but this effort engages the internal rotation component of the tensor fascia lata and gluteus medius muscles, internally rotating the thighs.

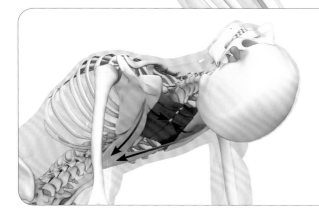

STEP 5 Contract the rhomboids and lower third of the trapezius to draw the scapulae toward the midline and the shoulders away from the neck. This frees the cervical spine to relax, the head to drop back, and the chest to open upward.

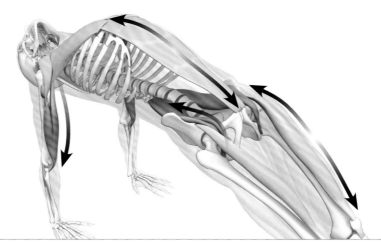

SUMMARY All of these steps conspire to stretch the entire front side of the body. The muscles at the tops of the feet that extend the toes and the tibialis anterior on the fronts of the lower legs stretch. The rectus femoris, although part of the contracting quadriceps, also stretches from the hips extending. This muscle eccentrically contracts in Purvottanasana as you straighten the knees. The psoas and its synergists of hip flexion lengthen. Preparatory facilitated stretches of these muscles help to extend the femurs and deepen the pose. The abdominals lengthen; however, you should gently engage them during this backbend to produce the abdominal "air bag" effect, protecting the lumbar spine from hyperextension. Extending the arms stretches the pectoralis major and anterior deltoids. Straightening the elbows stretches the biceps and brachialis muscles.

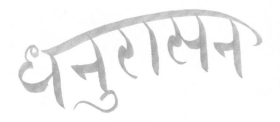

DHANURASANA

BOW POSE

IN DHANURASANA, WE CONNECT THE UPPER AND LOWER APPENDICULAR skeletons (the hands and the feet) to lever the axial skeleton (the spinal column) into extension. Grasping the ankles with the hands is a secondary action that contributes to the primary stretch of the front of the body.

The shoulders extend to lift the feet, with the arms forming the string of the bow. Lifting the arms and bending the elbows tightens the body of the bow—the femurs, pelvis, and trunk. The body of the bow stretches, resisting the action of the arms to form a bandha. Work toward extending the hips and straightening the knees; this pulls on the arms to further extend the spine. All of these actions combine to deepen and stabilize the posture. Facilitated stretches that create length in the fronts of the hips and shoulders, such as those described in the preparation, can be used to train these regions of the body for Dhanurasana.

Numerous subplots contribute to the final pose. For example, you can grip the ankles more firmly and then bend the elbows. Gripping tightly with the hands will recruit additional fibers in the muscles that flex the elbows—the biceps and brachialis. Bending the elbows and straightening the knees increases the stretch of the front of the body and the bend of the back of the body.

BASIC JOINT POSITIONS

- The shoulders extend.
- The elbows extend.
- The forearms pronate.
- The hips extend, internally rotate, and adduct.
- The knees flex.
- The ankles dorsiflex (extend).
- The trunk extends.

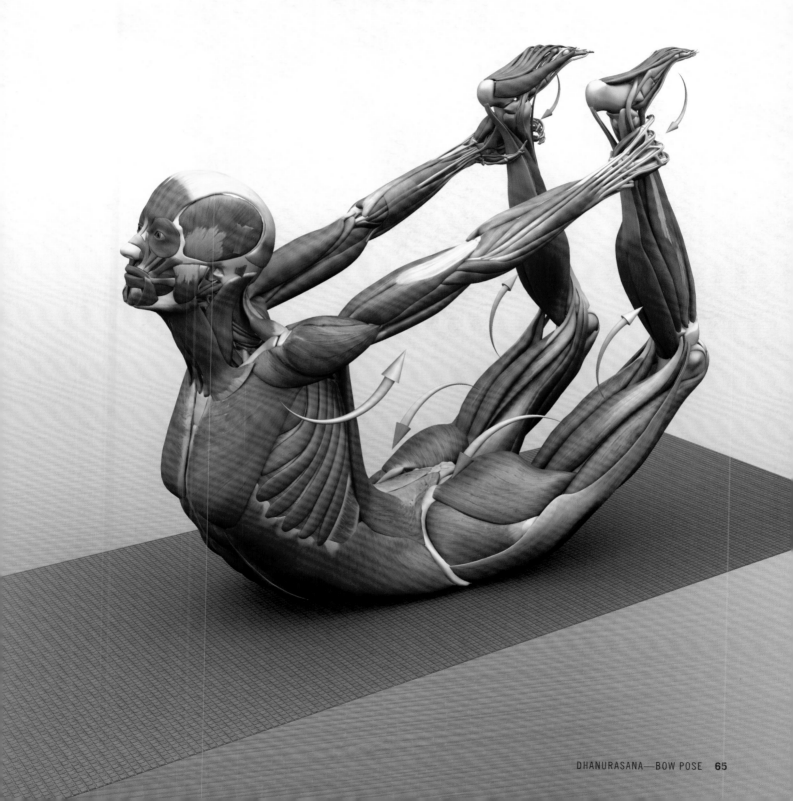

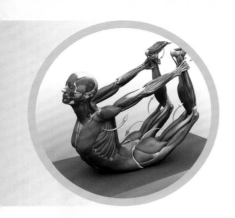

Dhanurasana Preparation

Lie on the stomach and bend the knees to grasp the ankles with the hands. Use a belt to reach the ankles if necessary. Squeeze the buttocks (gluteus maximus) to create the general shape of the pose, which includes extension of the spine and hips. Tighten the grip on the ankles and dorsiflex them to create a "lock" between the upper and lower extremities.

Try placing a bolster under the thighs. Then place the bolster under the lower chest, and feel how this changes the stretch. Finally, straighten the knees to lift the legs and arch the back. Ease out of the pose by bending the knees and lowering the legs to the floor. Then release your grip.

Prepare the shoulder and hip flexors separately using the isolated facilitated stretches shown here.

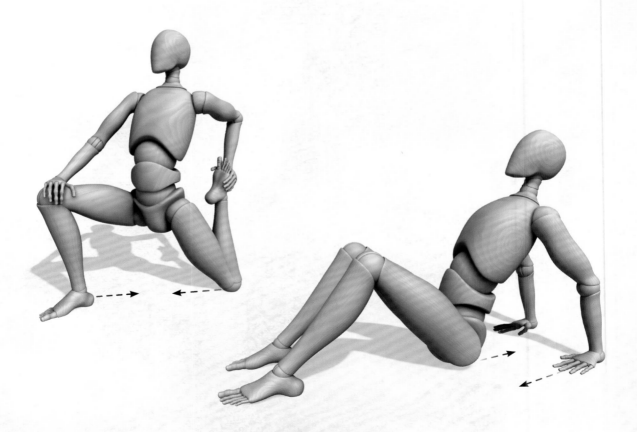

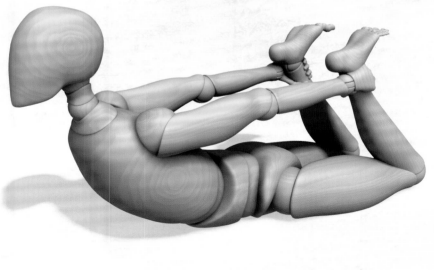

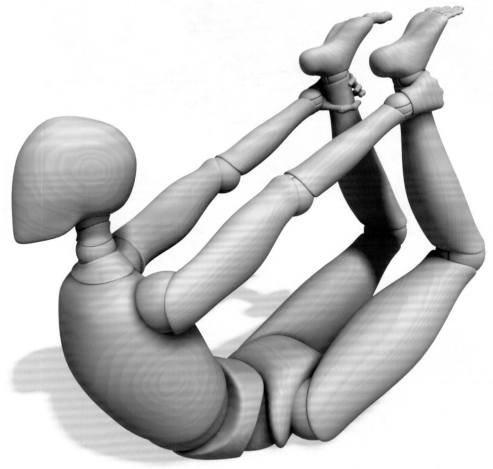

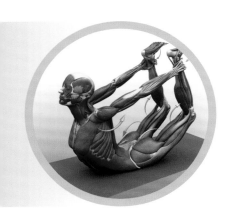

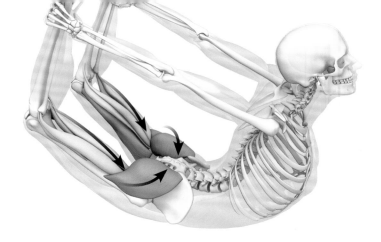

STEP 1 Engage the gluteus maximus to extend the hips. In the initial phase of the posture, use the hamstrings to bring the ankles within range of the hands so that you can hold them. Deepen the pose by activating the quadriceps to straighten the knees. Then co-activate the hamstrings and gluteus maximus to roll the pelvis back and down. The force that tilts the pelvis also helps to lift the back. Note that extending the hips with the gluteus maximus causes the knees to splay apart due to the external rotation component of this muscle. Contract the adductor magnus to draw the knees together and synergize extending the femurs. Additionally, press the outsides of the ankles against the hands to engage the tensor fascia lata and gluteus medius muscles, internally rotating the thighs.

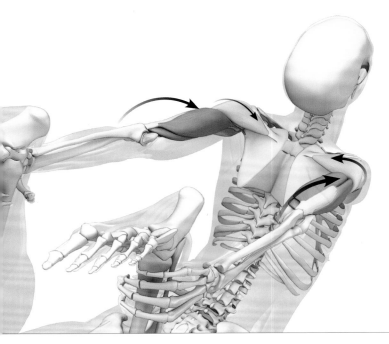

◀ **STEP 2** Engage the rhomboids to draw the shoulder blades toward the midline. Extend the upper arm bones (the humeri) up and back, away from the trunk. This activates the posterior portion of the deltoids. Before you go into the pose, lift one arm behind you and then reach around from the front with the other hand; you can feel the posterior deltoid contract on the back of the shoulder. Activate this muscle on both sides while in the pose to lift the arms. Engage the triceps to straighten the elbows. Note how the actions of the rhomboids, posterior deltoids, and triceps combine to lift the legs and deepen the stretch.

STEP 3 Extend the vertebral column by engaging the erector spinae and quadratus lumborum. Draw the shoulders away from the neck with the lower trapezius. When you extend the back, the spine curves more, loosening the string of the bow (the arms grasping the ankles). Activate the quadriceps to extend the knees. This re-tightens the string of the bow while maintaining the extension of the spine.

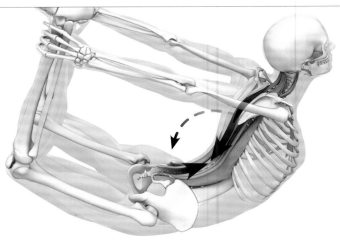

▶ **STEP 4** Engage the tibialis anterior and extensors hallucis and digitorum longus to dorsiflex the ankles; contract the peroneus longus and brevis muscles on the sides of the lower legs to evert them. These actions create a lock for the hands to more firmly grip the ankles.

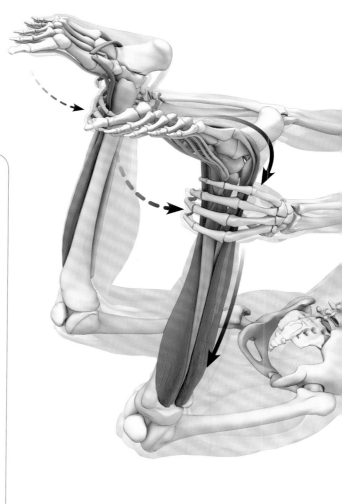

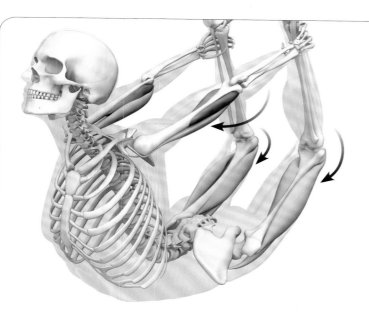

STEP 5 Once the spine is fully extended, bend the elbows by contracting the biceps and brachialis muscles while engaging the quadriceps to straighten the knees. These opposing forces create a bandha.

SUMMARY Note how each region of the body—the shoulders, elbows, wrists, and hands on the upper body; the hips, knees, and ankles on the lower body; and the muscles at the back of the trunk—all work together to stretch the entire front side of the body. Extending the upper extremities away from the back stretches the pectoralis major, the anterior deltoids, and the biceps and brachialis muscles. Arching the back stretches the rectus abdominis. Eccentrically contract the abdominals to engage the "air bag" effect. This aids to strengthen the abdominals while protecting the lower back. Extending the hips stretches the hip flexors, including the psoas and its synergists (the pectineus, adductors longus and brevis, sartorius, and rectus femoris).

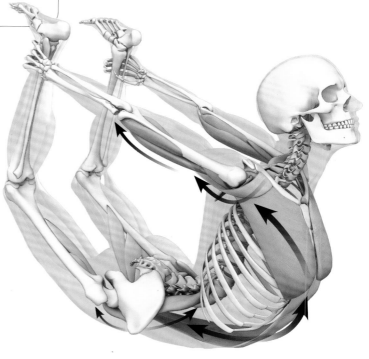

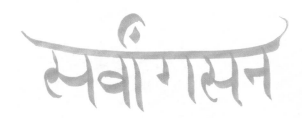

SETU BANDHA SARVANGASANA

BRIDGE POSE

SETU BANDHA SARVANGASANA COMBINES ARCHING THE BACK WITH EXTENDING the shoulders to lift the pelvis and torso. This pose places the heart lower than most of the trunk, creating a light inversion that improves the return of venous blood to the heart, thereby augmenting cardiac output. There may also be a temporary increase in parasympathetic outflow from the central nervous system, which can lower the heart rate. Accordingly, Bridge Pose shares many of the potential benefits of the conventional inversions, such as Headstand and Shoulder Stand. It can be used as an alternative by people with cervical spine pathology or contraindications that prevent them from doing other inverted postures.

Additionally, Setu Bandha stretches the flexor muscles at the front of the pelvis, including the psoas and its synergists. It can be done after the Psoas Awakening Series described in *The Key Poses of Yoga* to counterbalance vigorous activation of the hip flexors.

BASIC JOINT POSITIONS

- The shoulders extend and externally rotate.
- The elbows extend.
- The forearms supinate.

- The knees flex.
- The hips extend, internally rotate, and adduct.
- The trunk extends.

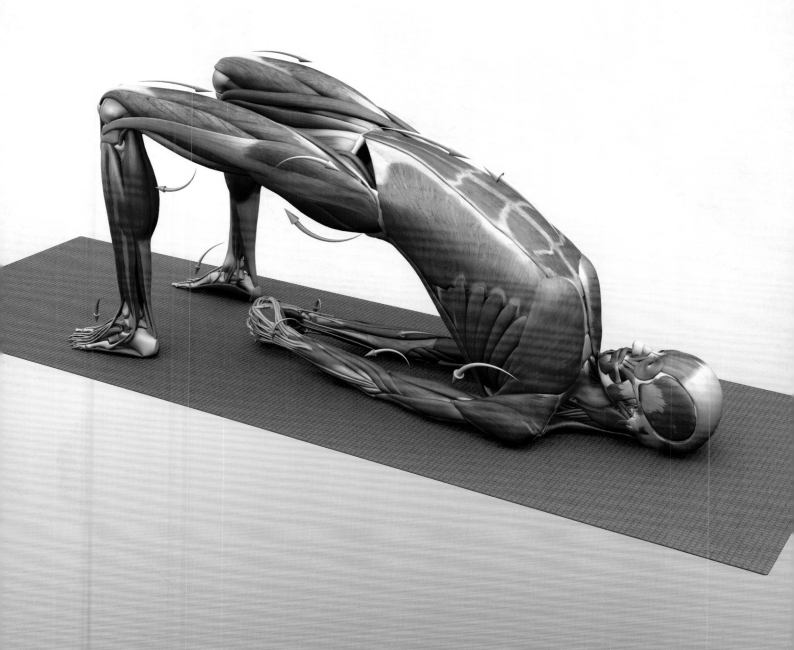

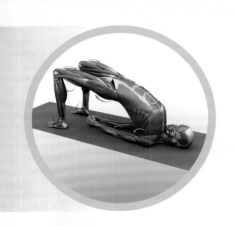

Setu Bandha Sarvangasana
Preparation

Begin by dividing the pose into its components—the actions of the pelvis, hips, and shoulder girdle. Practice the psoas and rectus femoris stretch shown here to prepare for extending the hips. Add a facilitated component as needed for a deeper stretch. Similarly, use the shoulder flexor stretch to prepare for extending the upper arms in the asana.

For the final pose, there are a variety of options to choose from. For example, try a supported variation by placing a block under the sacrum. Another option is to link the hands and feet with a belt or rope (Chatush Padasana). If you are flexible enough, grasp the ankles with the hands. You can also intertwine the fingers and extend the arms, pressing the little finger sides of the hands into the mat. Breathe deeply and open the chest while keeping the neck relaxed. Come out of the pose by releasing the arms and walking the feet out. Lower the torso onto the floor and rest there for a moment.

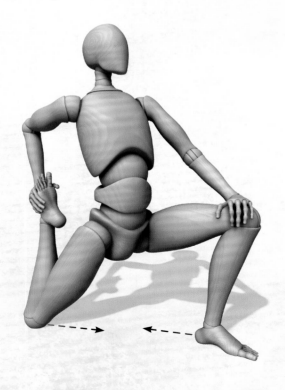

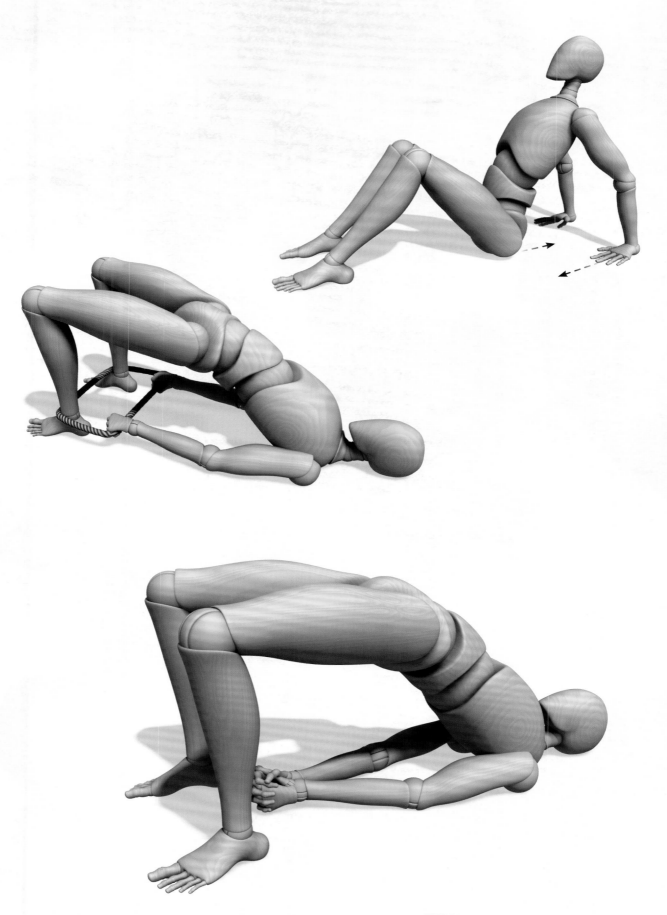

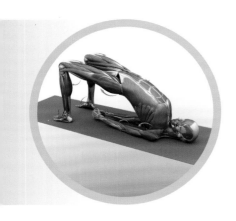

STEP 1 Tuck the tailbone under and draw the pelvis upward by contracting the gluteus maximus and hamstring muscles. We generally think of the hamstrings as flexors of the knees. However, these muscles can also move their origins on the ischial tuberosities of the pelvis. This can be used to lift the pelvis, as shown. The gluteus minimus is a synergist of hip extension and aids the gluteus maximus when the hips are in this position. The more posterior portion of the gluteus medius also assists in extending the hips.

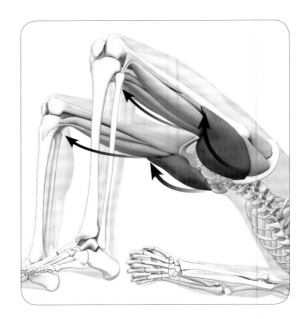

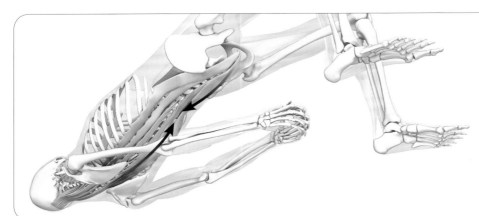

STEP 2 Arch the back by contracting the erector spinae and quadratus lumborum. Engage these muscles along with the gluteals to create lumbopelvic rhythm, whereby the pelvis tilts into retroversion while the lumbar spine extends.

▶ **STEP 3** Once you have lifted the pelvis, relax the hamstrings and activate the quadriceps to deepen the pose. Remember that the quadriceps extend the knees. Because the feet are fixed on the mat, attempting to straighten the knees actually lifts the torso.

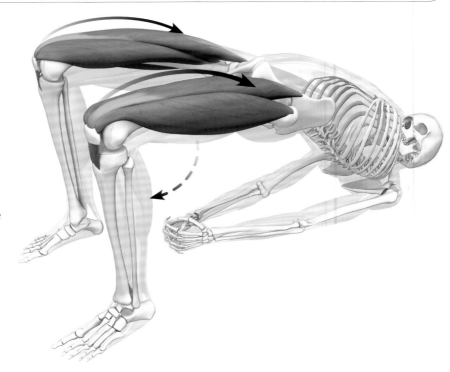

STEP 4 Extend the shoulders by contracting the posterior deltoid and teres major muscles. The latissimus dorsi (not pictured here) initiates this action; however, when the arms are in this position, the latissimus dorsi is unable to add much additional extension. This is known as active insufficiency.

Contract the triceps to extend the elbows. Supinate the forearms by interlacing the fingers and then gently turning the palms upward. Externally rotate the shoulders with the infraspinatus and teres minor muscles. The posterior deltoids contribute to this action. Note how supinating the forearms also synergizes externally rotating the shoulders. Finally, adduct the scapulae toward the midline with the rhomboids and draw the shoulders away from the neck with the lower third of the trapezius. These actions work together to open the chest.

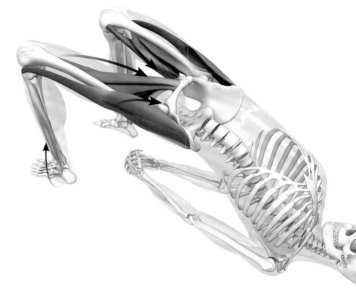

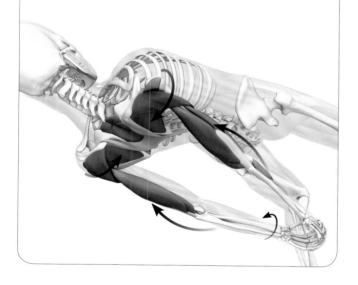

STEP 5 Although contracting the gluteus maximus has the beneficial effect of extending the hips, it also has the undesirable effect of rolling the thighs outward, causing them to splay apart. We want to retain the beneficial effects while using other muscles to counteract the splaying of the thighs. To do this, activate the peroneus longus and brevis on the sides of the lower legs to press the balls of the feet into the mat. Then attempt to draw the feet apart. This engages the tensor fascia lata and gluteus medius (abductors of the hips). The feet are fixed on the mat and so the legs will not actually abduct, but the thighs roll inward due to the internal rotation component of these muscles. Finally, draw the knees together by contracting the adductor group of muscles on the insides of the thighs. The most posterior of these, the adductor magnus, also synergizes the gluteus maximus to extend the hips.

▶ **SUMMARY** All of these actions conspire to stretch the pectorals, anterior deltoids, biceps, and coracobrachialis muscles on the front of the chest and arms. Extending the trunk lengthens the rectus abdominis. Eccentrically contract these muscles to produce the abdominal "air bag" effect, thereby protecting the lumbar spine from hyperextension. Drawing the shoulder blades toward the midline stretches the serratus anterior muscles. Extending the hips lengthens the psoas and its synergists of hip flexion: the pectineus, the adductors longus and brevis, and the sartorius. The rectus femoris also stretches. This muscle eccentrically contracts when you straighten the knees, as in Step 3.

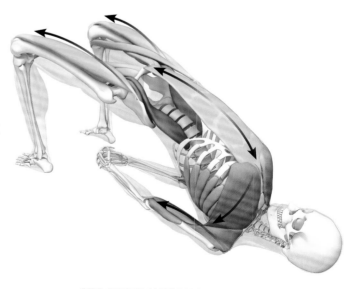

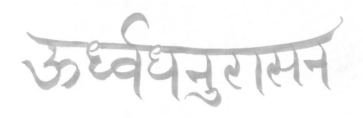

URDHVA DHANURASANA

UPWARD FACING BOW POSE

IN URDHVA DHANURASANA THE DIRECTION OF THE SHOULDERS SHIFTS TO a position of forward or frontal flexion (compared with the previous poses in this series, which extend the shoulders away from the back). Thus the shoulder stretch changes in this pose: the muscles that extend the arms are now lengthening. The arch of the torso is raised higher, taking the front of the body into a deeper stretch. The muscles at the front of the pelvis lengthen more because the hips are in greater extension. Firmly extending the elbows and the knees creates subplots to the main story of this pose, deepening it. The hands and feet are fixed to the mat, so the energy of straightening the arms and legs is transferred to the trunk, indirectly extending the back and hips and stretching the front of the body.

BASIC JOINT POSITIONS

- The shoulders flex and abduct.
- The elbows extend.
- The forearms pronate.
- The wrists extend.
- The hips extend, internally rotate, and adduct.
- The knees extend.
- The feet pronate.
- The trunk extends.

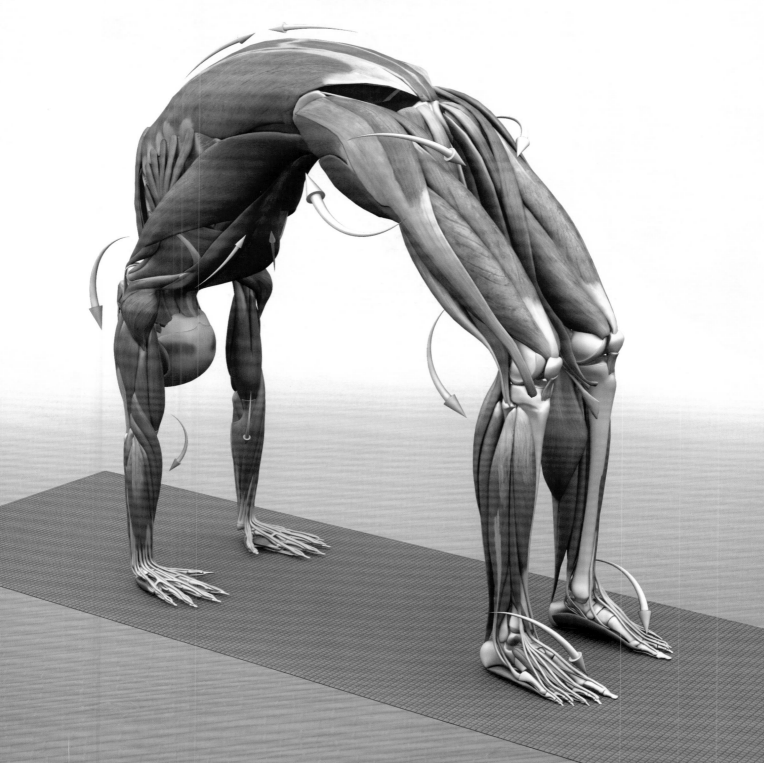

URDHVA DHANURASANA—UPWARD FACING BOW POSE **77**

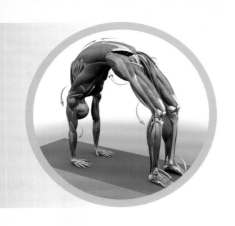

Urdhva Dhanurasana Preparation

Lie supine (belly up) on the mat. Bend the knees so that the lower legs are at right angles to the floor and place the feet about hip-width distance apart. You may use a belt to catch the ankles with the hands. Then engage the hamstrings and gluteus maximus to lift the pelvis and extend the hips. This is a good place to pause to gain flexibility. Then add the arms. Place the hands just above the shoulders, as shown. Press the palms down evenly while arching the pelvis upward. Contract the adductor muscles to draw the knees toward each other and turn the thighs inward. Ease the body up to place the top of the head on the mat. Draw the shoulder blades toward the midline of the spine and expand the chest. If you are new to the pose, pause here for a moment and then come out.

When you have the strength, press the hands into the mat and extend the elbows to lift the trunk, at the same time straightening the knees. Hold the final pose for several smooth and even breaths. Carefully ease out by bending the elbows, walking the feet away from the hands, and bending the knees to place the back on the ground.

Isolate and lengthen the shoulder extensors using the chair stretch shown here. You can turn this into a facilitated stretch by intermittently pressing the elbows down onto the seat of the chair to stimulate the relaxation response.

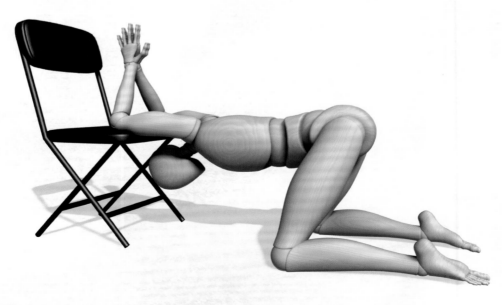

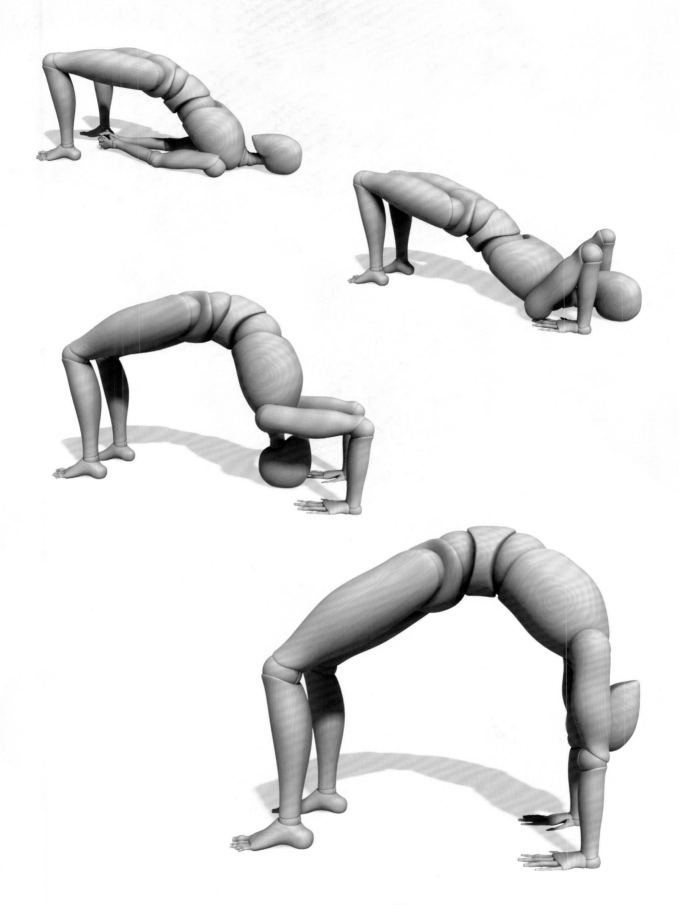

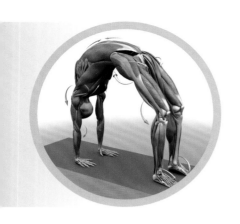

STEP 1 Temporarily activate the hamstrings to extend the hips. The cue for this action is to attempt to drag the soles of the feet toward the pelvis. The feet are glued to the mat, so the force of the contraction is transmuted to lifting the hips. Then engage the gluteus maximus, medius, and minimus by squeezing the buttocks to extend the femurs and retrovert the pelvis. A beneficial effect of contracting the gluteus maximus is the downward tilt of the pelvis, which protects against hyperextension of the lumbar spine. A side effect of contracting the gluteus maximus is external rotation of the femurs. This causes the legs to splay apart. In Urdhva Dhanurasana we want to maintain the beneficial effect of engaging the gluteus maximus while counteracting the undesirable effect of externally rotating and splaying the femurs apart. Step 6 explains how to do this. Contract the adductor magnus to draw the knees together. This muscle also synergizes the gluteals in extending the hips.

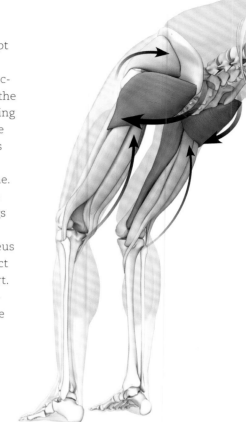

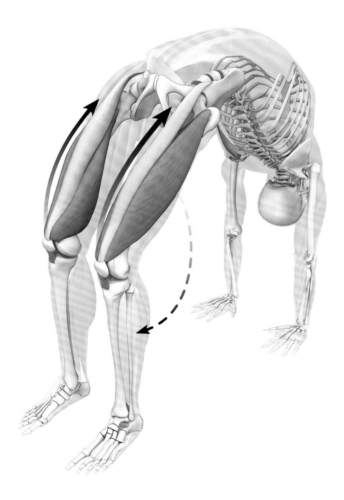

◄ **STEP 2** Engage the quadriceps to straighten the knees. This indirectly extends the hips because the feet are glued to the mat. They cannot "kick out" in front, so the quadriceps act like a hydraulic lift to raise the pelvis. Notice the rectus femoris portion of the quadriceps here in light blue. This muscle crosses the hip and knee joints, moving both when it contracts; thus it is polyarticular. (The other parts of the quadriceps only cross the knee and are monoarticular). The rectus femoris tilts the pelvis forward, anteverting it. This rotational effect on the pelvis helps to extend the spine, and the retroversion helps to protect against hyperextension.

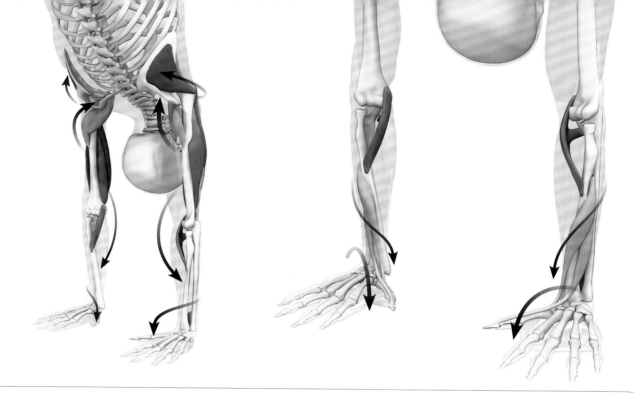

STEP 3 Pronate the forearms to press the hands into the mat, spreading the weight from the mounds of the index fingers across the rest of the palms. Contract the triceps to straighten the elbows. Note that the long head of the triceps attaches to the scapula. Firmly engaging this muscle aids to rotate the scapula away from the humerus and prevents impingement on the acromion process. This gives more room to flex the arms above the head. Activate the infraspinatus and teres minor muscles to externally rotate the shoulders, creating a helical action down the arms and through the elbows. A cue for this is to imagine rotating the hands outward while they are fixed on the mat, as if you were washing a window.

Engage the anterior deltoids to flex the shoulders further, drawing the trunk deeper into the pose from the arms. To gain awareness of this muscle before going into the pose, raise one arm in front of you and feel the front of the shoulder with the other hand. This is the anterior deltoid contracting. To activate this muscle while in the pose, attempt to "scrub" the hands toward the feet. Experience how this deepens the asana.

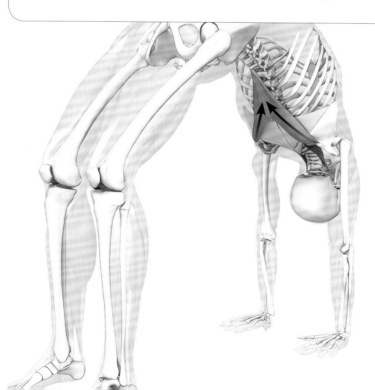

STEP 4 Draw the shoulder blades toward the midline by engaging the rhomboids. Note that the scapulae rotate outward when the arms are above the head. Use the lower third of the trapezius to depress the scapulae and draw the shoulders away from the neck. The rhomboids and trapezius muscles combine to exert a tethering affect on the shoulder blades, stabilizing them.

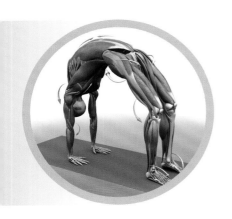

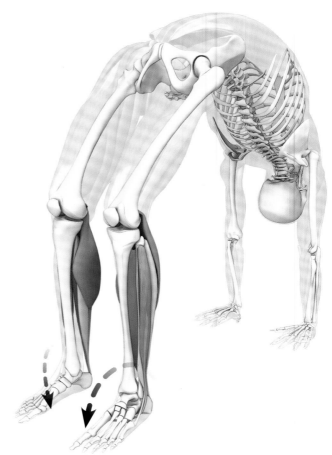

STEP 5 Plantar flex the ankles and press the weight into the soles of the feet, activating the gastrocnemius and soleus muscles. Begin by pressing the heels into the mat, and then evert the ankles to distribute the weight evenly into the balls of the feet. This engages the peroneus longus and brevis muscles on the sides of the lower legs. These actions secure the feet on the mat and are the first steps in addressing the splaying of the thighs caused by the gluteus maximus (described in Step 1).

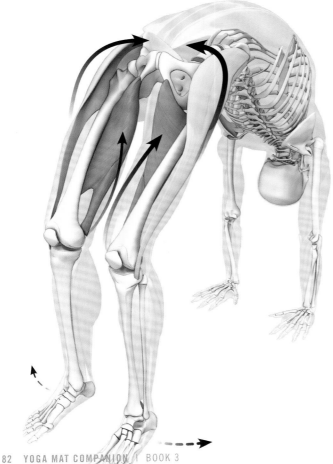

STEP 6 Contract the tensor fascia lata and gluteus medius muscles to internally rotate the hips, counteracting the external rotation forces of the hip extensors—the gluteus maximus and adductor magnus. A cue for this is to maintain the feet well fixed on the mat, and then attempt to "scrub" them apart (abduction). Because the feet won't move, the thighs will roll inward (internal rotation is one action of the tensor fascia lata and gluteus medius). Then contract the adductor group to draw the knees toward the midline. You can gain awareness of the adductors in the preparatory phase of the pose by placing a block between the knees and squeezing it.

▶ **STEP 7** Urdhva Dhanurasana stretches the hip flexors, including the psoas, pectineus, adductors longus and brevis, sartorius, and rectus femoris. The abdominals also stretch in this pose. Gently contract them to engage the abdominal "air bag" effect, which helps to protect the lumbar spine. This eccentric contraction creates a facilitated stretch of the abdominals, so that they lengthen on relaxation as a result of stimulating the Golgi tendon organ.

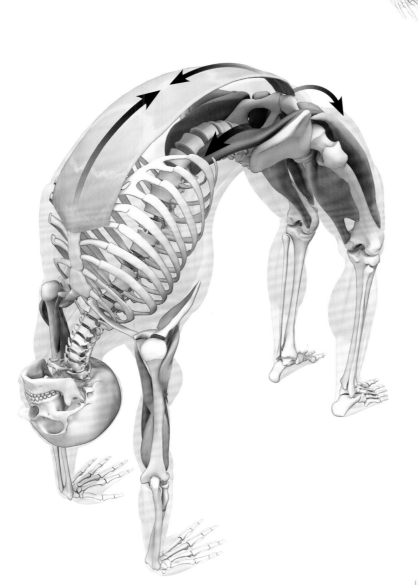

SUMMARY The shoulders flex in Urdhva Dhanurasana, stretching the muscles that extend the shoulders. These include the posterior deltoids, the latissimus dorsi, part of the pectoralis major, and the coracobrachialis. Extending the elbows stretches the biceps and brachialis muscles.

एकपादविपरीतदंडासन

EKA PADA VIPARITA DANDASANA

ONE-LEGGED INVERTED STAFF POSE

EKA PADA VIPARITA DANDASANA IS ONE OF THE MOST ADVANCED BACKBENDING poses and therefore requires extensive preparation. There are several stories or foci of the pose, including an inversion, a backbend, and the splits. The hip of the lifted leg flexes and the knee extends as in Hanumanasana. The hip of the leg that remains on the floor extends, with the knee initially flexing and then straightening to deepen the pose, as in Urdhva Dhanurasana. Then there is the balance component, with the forearms and standing leg forming a tripod to support the inverted torso. Accordingly, one should be competent in inversions, backbends, and the splits to perform Eka Pada Viparita Dandasana.

Each component of this pose can be deconstructed into smaller parts that contribute to the whole. Preparation and training should focus on facilitated stretching of the hip flexors, hip extensors, and hamstrings, as detailed in the section on Hanumanasana. You can also apply several preparatory stretches for gaining mobility in the shoulders.

The grip on the ankle serves as a stabilizer, and the elbows act as a fulcrum for opening the upper back. The leg on the floor can be extended at the knee to indirectly lift the pelvis and deepen the backbend. The leg in the air depends mainly on the strength of the hip and knee extensors to straighten, as well as on the length in the antagonist muscles at the back of the leg to allow this movement. If you have created sufficient length in your hamstrings and gluteals, you can flex the hip and extend the knee with much less effort than if these muscles are tight.

BASIC JOINT POSITIONS

- The shoulders flex.
- The elbows flex and the forearms supinate.
- The hip of the leg that remains on the floor extends, internally rotates, and adducts.
- The knee of the same leg flexes.
- The trunk extends.
- The raised-leg hip flexes.
- The raised-leg knee extends.
- The raised-leg ankle dorsiflexes and the toes extend.

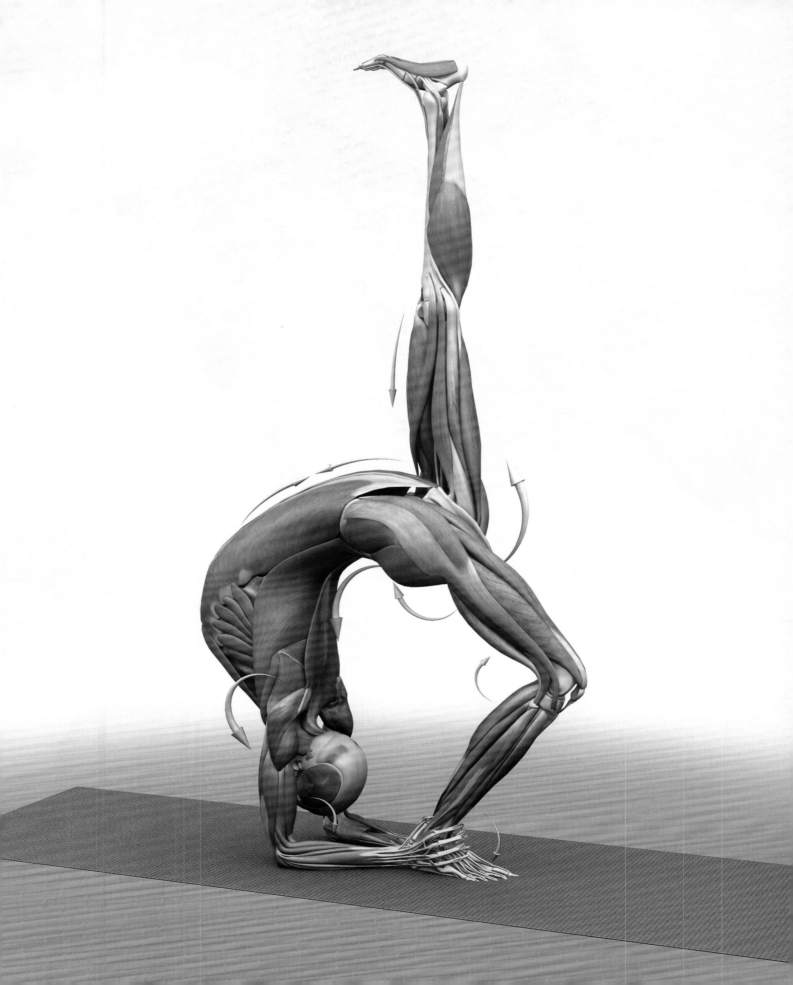

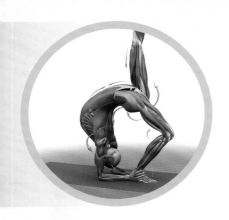

Eka Pada Viparita Dandasana Preparation

Begin in Urdhva Dhanurasana; then place the head on the floor inside the palms. This is Dwi Pada Viparita Dandasana. Press up by engaging the buttocks and straightening the knees. This is a good place to pause when learning the pose. Let the brain integrate this position before moving on.

When you are stable in Dwi Pada Viparita Dandasana, walk one foot toward the midline to create the apex of the triangle. This is the foot you will eventually link with the upper extremities. Lift the other foot off the floor by flexing the hip to draw the knee toward the torso. Hold this position for a few breaths and then come down. As you gain confidence in the pose, you can begin to straighten the lifted knee by contracting the quadriceps. To advance further, use a belt to grasp the ankle and lift the head off the floor, opening the shoulders. With great flexibility, you may link the ankle with the hands as shown.

Ease out of the asana by placing the foot back on the floor and lifting up into a partial Urdhva Dhanurasana; then carefully lower the trunk down onto the mat. Prepare the hip flexors and extensors using the chair-assisted Hanumanasana stretch.

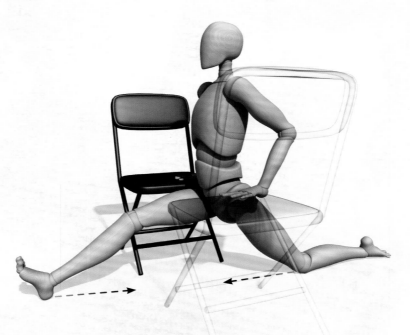

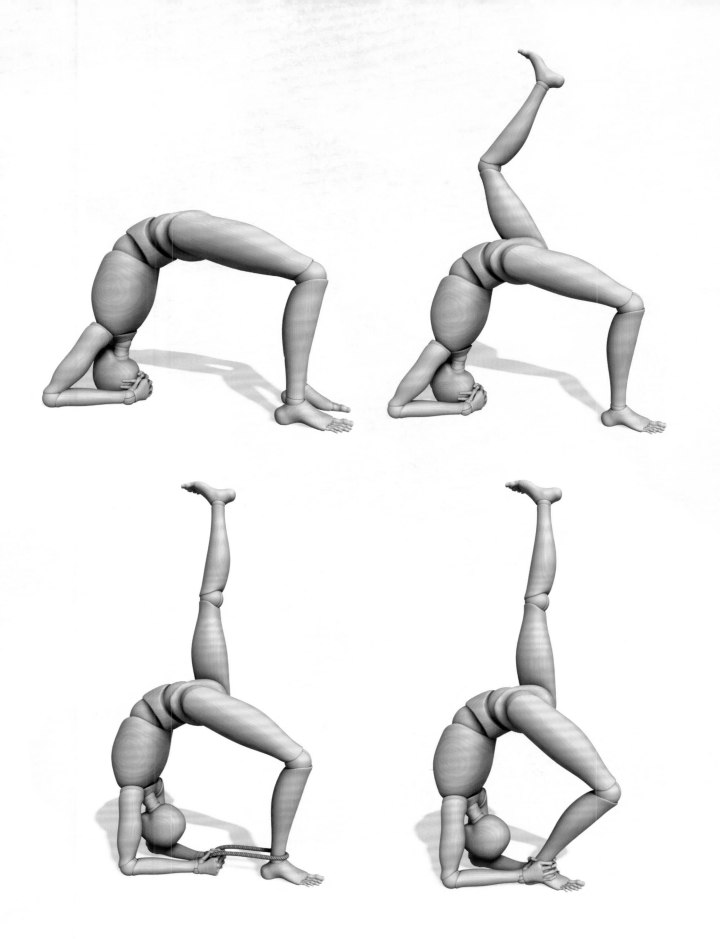

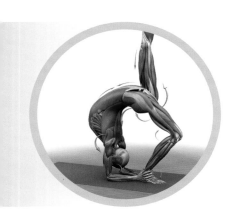

STEP 1 Extend the back with the erector spinae and quadratus lumborum, and gently lift the head toward the leg. Draw the torso toward the foot by activating the anterior deltoids. The back muscles synergize with the anterior deltoids, levator scapulae, and upper trapezius to deepen the pose. Contract the biceps and brachialis to bend the elbows. Note how this draws you closer to the feet, opening the chest. Maintain the position of the chest, and then contract the triceps to press the forearms into the mat, bringing the upper arm bones perpendicular to the floor.

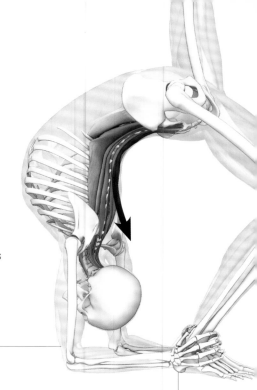

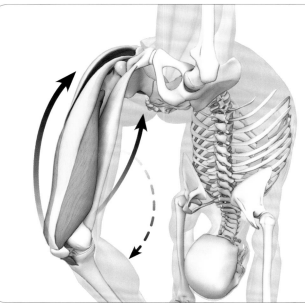

STEP 2 Activate the quadriceps to partially extend the knee and lift the pelvis higher. Because the foot is fixed on the mat and cannot kick out, the force of contracting the quadriceps lifts the pelvis. The adductor magnus draws the knee toward the midline and assists in extending the hip.

STEP 3 Engage the serratus anterior and trapezius to externally rotate the scapulae. Roll the shoulders outward by contracting the infraspinatus and teres minor muscles, and tilt the head back from the cervical spine.

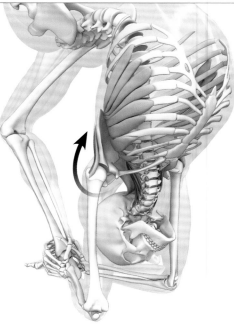

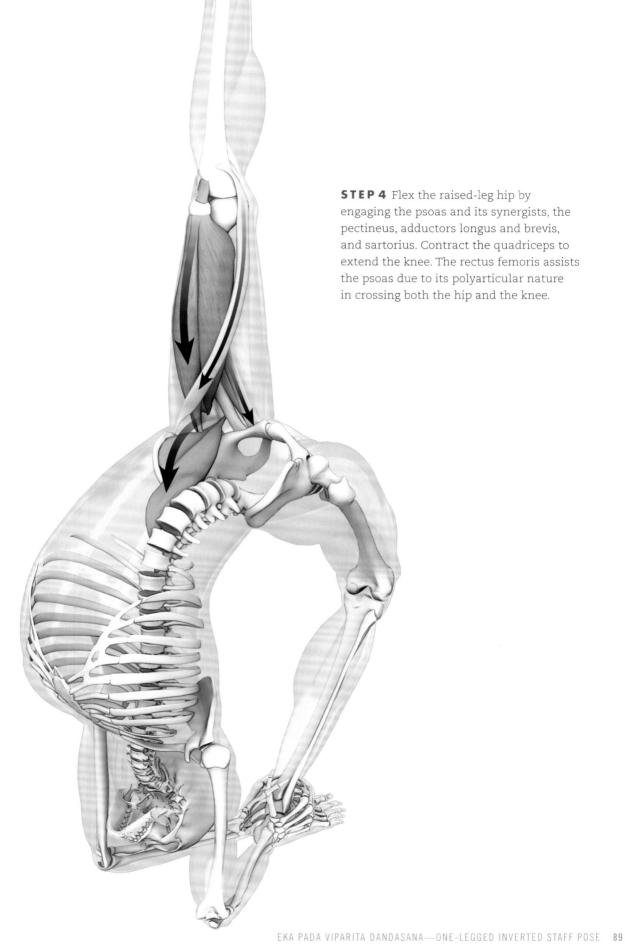

STEP 4 Flex the raised-leg hip by engaging the psoas and its synergists, the pectineus, adductors longus and brevis, and sartorius. Contract the quadriceps to extend the knee. The rectus femoris assists the psoas due to its polyarticular nature in crossing both the hip and the knee.

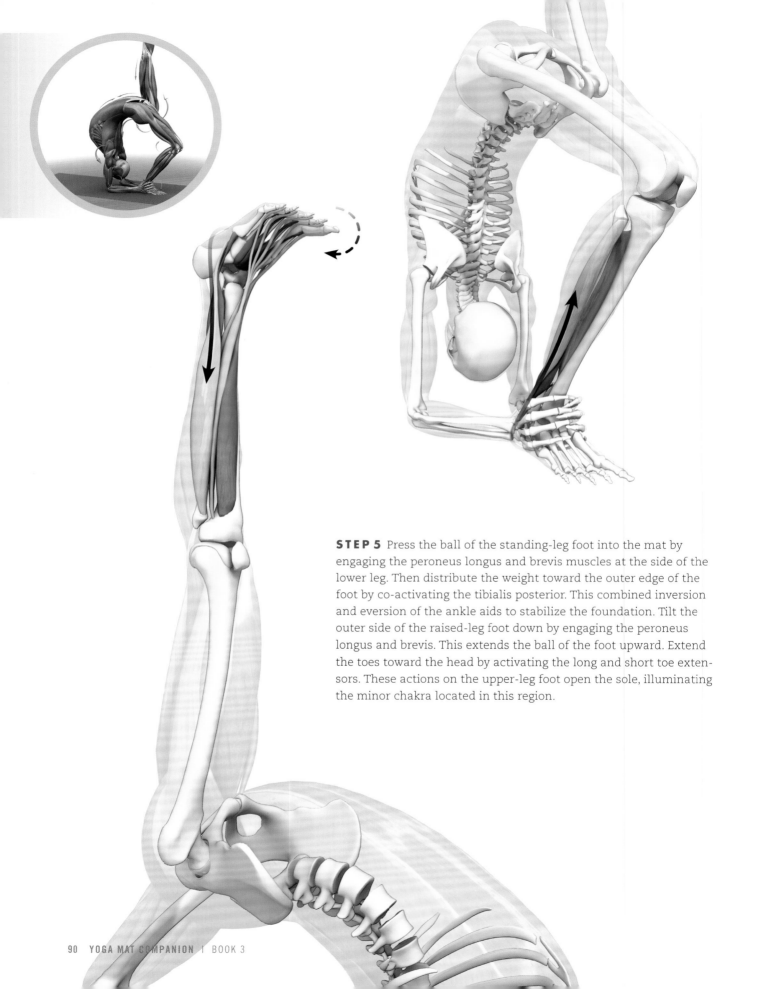

STEP 5 Press the ball of the standing-leg foot into the mat by engaging the peroneus longus and brevis muscles at the side of the lower leg. Then distribute the weight toward the outer edge of the foot by co-activating the tibialis posterior. This combined inversion and eversion of the ankle aids to stabilize the foundation. Tilt the outer side of the raised-leg foot down by engaging the peroneus longus and brevis. This extends the ball of the foot upward. Extend the toes toward the head by activating the long and short toe extensors. These actions on the upper-leg foot open the sole, illuminating the minor chakra located in this region.

SUMMARY Raising the leg stretches the hip extensors, including the gluteus maximus and adductor magnus. Flexing the hip and extending the knee triangulates the hamstrings, stretching them from both their origin and their insertions. Extending the knee and dorsiflexing the foot stretches the gastrocnemius. The lower-side hip flexors stretch, including the psoas, pectineus, and adductors longus and brevis. The rectus femoris lengthens and eccentrically contracts. The latissimus dorsi, teres major, posterior deltoids, and pectoralis major (the sternocostal portion) all lengthen from the deep extension of the shoulders. The abdominals stretch, as with all poses that extend the trunk. Gently eccentrically contract the abdominals to engage the abdominal "air bag" effect, and activate the pubococcygeus muscle to nutate the pelvis and protect the spine.

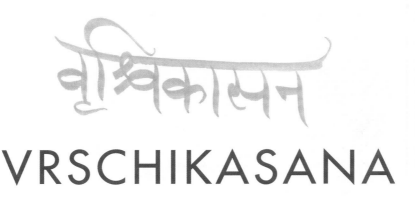

VRSCHIKASANA

SCORPION POSE

THREE SEPARATE STORIES TAKE PLACE SIMULTANEOUSLY IN VRSCHIKASANA: a backbend, an arm balance, and an inversion. Deconstruct the pose into these elements and then work on each separately. For example, use isolated facilitated stretching to develop flexibility in the hips and shoulders. Work on the subplots of the inversion and arm balance components by practicing poses such as Pincha Mayurasana. Then combine the parts to create the whole that is Scorpion Pose.

Observe the principles of physics and biomechanics operating in the arm balance. In the ideal position, the body weight "perches" on the humerus bones, so that the direction of gravity—the mechanical axis—aligns with the anatomical axes of the humeri. The muscular stabilizers of the shoulders also play an important role. Optimal stability requires that you engage each layer of the shoulder musculature from deep to superficial. The deep muscles include the rhomboids, which secure the scapulae, and the rotator cuff, which stabilizes the glenohumeral joints. The superficial shoulder muscles include the trapezius, deltoids, and pectorals. All of these combine to steady the shoulder girdle, which is the key to balance in this inversion. Outwardly rotating the humeri also creates ligamentotaxis by tightening the capsule and other fibrous structures to fix the shoulders in place.

Remember that aligning gravity against the long axes of the bones uses mechanical strength to support the body weight. Neither alignment of the bones nor ligamentotaxis requires muscular energy to exert its effect once the bones are brought into place. Accordingly, use the muscles to position the body in a manner that allows you to access these more effortless phenomena.

BASIC JOINT POSITIONS

- The shoulders flex.
- The elbows flex.
- The forearms pronate.
- The trunk extends.

- The hips extend, internally rotate, and adduct.
- The knees flex.
- The ankles plantar flex.
- The toes flex.

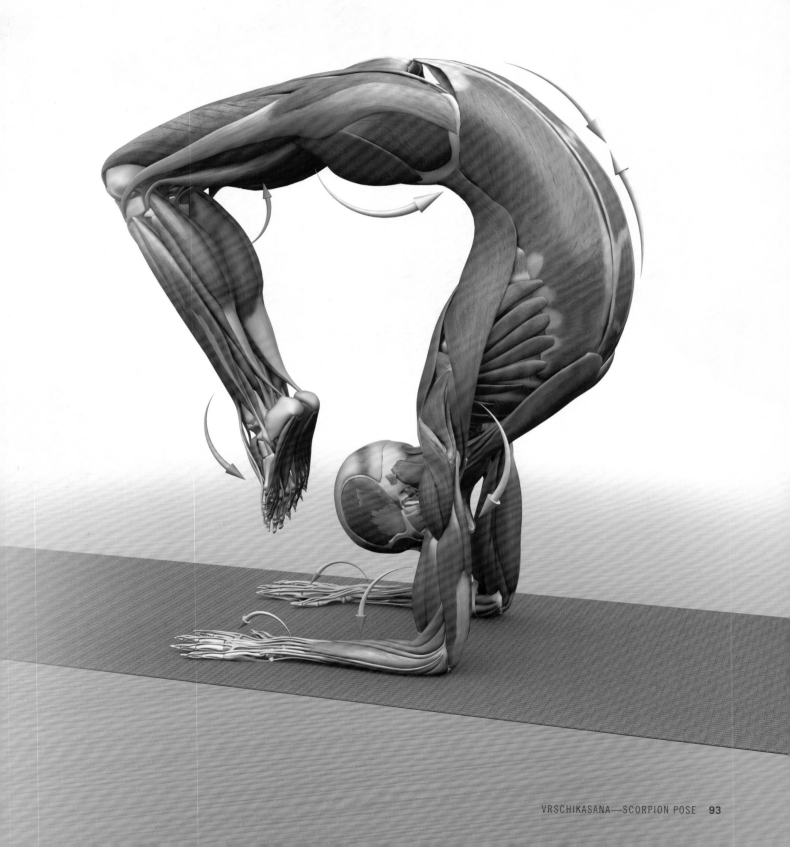

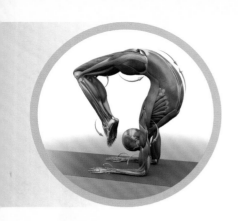

Vrschikasana Preparation

Deconstruct the pose and use isolated facilitated stretches to improve flexibility in the shoulders and hips. Practice Pincha Mayurasana against a wall to gain confidence with the inversion component of the posture. Once you feel comfortable there, begin to move the foundation formed by the forearms away from the wall, allowing the knees to bend and the feet to eventually drop over to touch the wall, as shown. At the same time, press down through the forearms and hands to lift up and out of the shoulders.

Next, place a chair between you and the wall. Carefully walk the feet down onto the back of the chair, and then press the pelvis upward by extending the hips and the knees. As you gain flexibility, you may walk the feet down the back of the chair and onto the seat, again extending the back of the body and lifting up from the shoulders. Then walk the feet in closer to the head, toward the edge of the chair, and eventually hook the toes over the chair edge. Finally, rest the soles of the feet on top of the head.

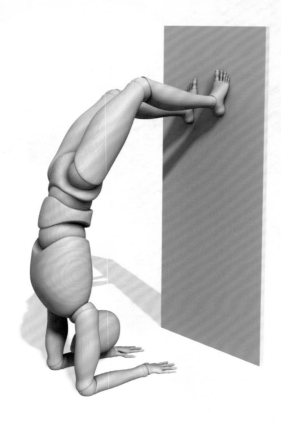

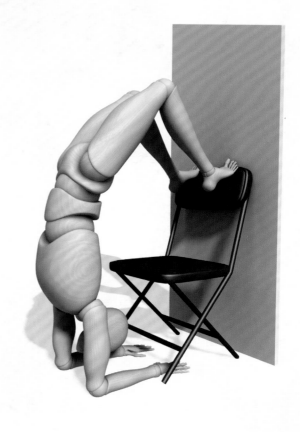

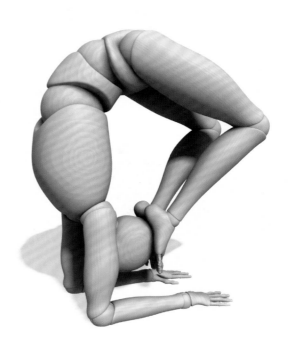

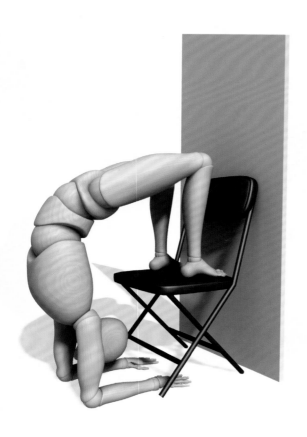

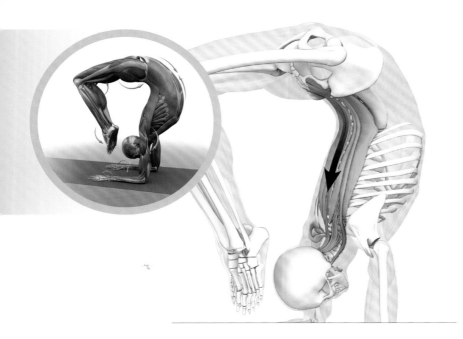

◀ STEP 1 Extend the spine by contracting the deep back extensors, including the erector spinae and quadratus lumborum muscles. Note the coupled movements and joint rhythm between the spine arching, the pelvis tilting forward (anteverting), and the femurs extending. The actions of the erector spinae and quadratus lumborum combine with the spine to connect the shoulder girdle and pelvis, creating the form of a scorpion.

STEP 2 Extend the hips by engaging the gluteus maximus, minimus, and posterior medius. Fibers from the gluteus maximus draw the femurs into external rotation, splaying the knees apart. Stretching the psoas also pulls the femurs into external rotation. Ideally, the femurs should project straight out from the hips toward parallel. This position requires flexibility in the fronts of the hips and strength in hip adduction and internal rotation. Activate the adductor magnus muscles to draw the knees together. Then imagine pressing the sides of the knees outward against a resistance. This engages the tensor fascia lata and the more anterior fibers of the gluteus medius, aiding to internally rotate the thighs.

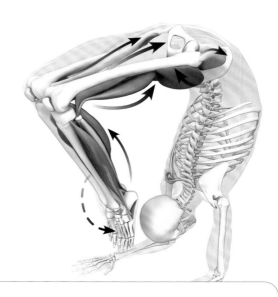

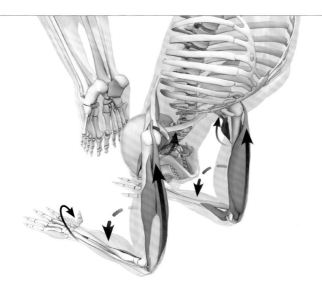

STEP 3 Contract the pronator teres and quadratus muscles of the forearms to press the palms of the hands into the floor, starting at the mounds of the index fingers. Spread the fingers and lightly grip the mat. Contract the triceps to bring the elbows into a right angle, so that the anatomical axes of the humerus bones align with the mechanical axis of gravity, aiding to support the weight of the body. Note that the long head of the triceps also crosses the shoulder joint and attaches to the lower part of the socket. This enables the triceps to act as a muscular stabilizer of the shoulder joint, synergizing the other stabilizers, including the rotator cuff. Draw the shoulders forward away from the hands, as if lifting the hands over the head. This engages the anterior deltoids, levator scapulae, and upper trapezius.

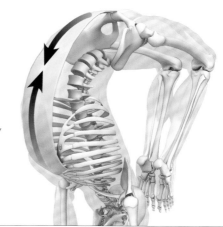

▶ **STEP 4** Gently contract the abdominals to engage the "air bag" effect. Notice how the rectus abdominis originates from the ribcage and inserts on the front middle of the pelvis at the pubic symphysis. Drawing these regions toward each other tilts the pelvis back into retroversion and eases off some of the lumbar hyperextension. Add to this protective effect by simultaneously engaging mula bandha, through the Kegel maneuver. This contracts the pubococcygeus muscle and nutates the sacrum within the iliac bones.

◀ **STEP 5** Engage the serratus anterior and trapezius muscles to rotate the scapulae outward and lift the torso upwards from the shoulders. Notice how this places the glenoid process (the shoulder socket) over the head of the humerus (the ball of the shoulder joint). This position supports the torso on the shoulders. Stabilize the head of the humerus in the socket by engaging the rotator cuff muscles, including the infraspinatus and teres minor. A cue for this is to rotate the shoulders externally. This has the added benefit of tightening the shoulder capsule, as well as the inferior glenohumeral ligament, which is the main ligamentous stabilizer of the shoulder in this position. This is an example of using ligamentotaxis to further stabilize the pose.

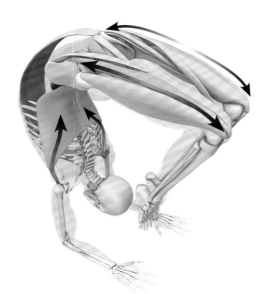

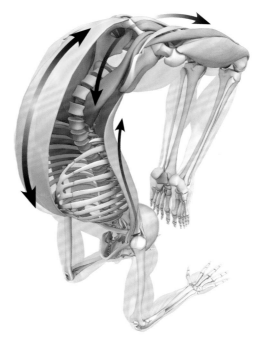

SUMMARY Vrschikasana combines an arm balance, backbend, and inversion to produce the form of a scorpion. Flexing the knees stretches the quadriceps. Extending the hips stretches the psoas, pectineus, and adductors longus and brevis; the sartorius and rectus femoris also lengthen. Extending the trunk stretches the abdominals, which we eccentrically contract to protect the lumbar spine. Flexing the shoulders lengthens the latissimus dorsi, the posterior deltoids, sternoclavicular portions of the pectoralis major, the coracobrachialis, and the biceps. Pronating the forearms stretches the supinator and biceps muscles.

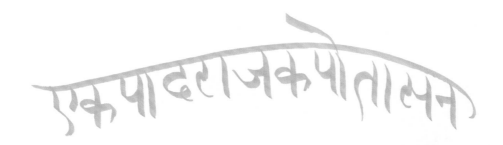

EKA PADA RAJA KAPOTASANA

PIGEON POSE

THREE STORIES TAKE PLACE SIMULTANEOUSLY IN EKA PADA RAJA KAPOTASANA. The front hip flexes, abducts, and externally rotates while the back hip extends, adducts, and internally rotates. The back extends. The opposing actions in the hips create a tethering force across the pelvis. Engaging the hip muscles that produce these opposing actions transmits a force across the sacroiliac ligaments, tightening them. This process, known as ligamentotaxis, aids to stabilize the pelvis. Deconstruct the pose into its elemental movements. Then determine where the blockages are. For example, the forward hip rotates outward, so it will be limited by tightness in the muscles that rotate the hip inward—the gluteus medius and tensor fascia lata. Identify, isolate, and use facilitated stretching to create length in these internal hip rotators. This releases the femur bones to turn outward. A converse process applies to the muscles of the back hip.

Find leverage points where you can use the connection between the upper and lower extremities to deepen the pose. For example, when you pull on the back foot with the hand, the back extends. Similarly, pressing into the mat and attempting to scrub backward with the other hand opens the chest forward. Note how these components interrelate in the final pose.

BASIC JOINT POSITIONS

- The forward-leg hip flexes, abducts, and externally rotates.
- The forward-leg knee flexes.
- The back-leg hip extends, internally rotates, and adducts.
- The back-leg knee flexes.
- The trunk extends.

- The shoulder of the arm that grasps the foot flexes and the elbow flexes.
- The shoulder of the arm that remains on the floor extends.
- The same-arm elbow extends and the forearm pronates.

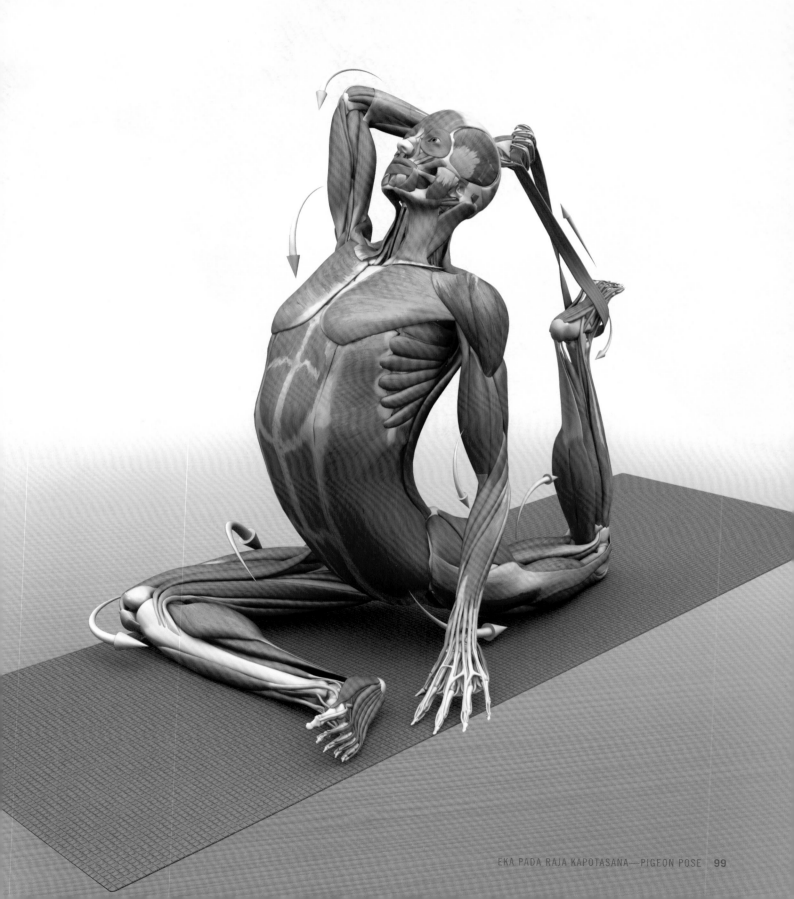

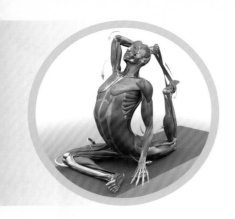

Eka Pada Raja
Kapotasana Preparation

In this preparatory series, begin by deconstructing the pose into constituent parts. First cradle the forward leg in the arms to stretch the internal rotators of the hip. Use facilitated stretching as necessary. Always support the knee in this type of action, and maintain it as a hinge joint to protect the cartilage and ligaments. If you cannot bring the leg into this position, then simply hold the foot and knee with the hands to develop flexibility. Release the stretch. Next, go into a lunge. Engage the back-leg gluteals and bend the front knee to deepen the stretch of the back hip flexors.

Once you attain a comfortable level of flexibility, combine the actions of the hips from the lunge and cradle stretch and loop a belt around the back foot as shown. The final touch is to grasp the back foot with the hands.

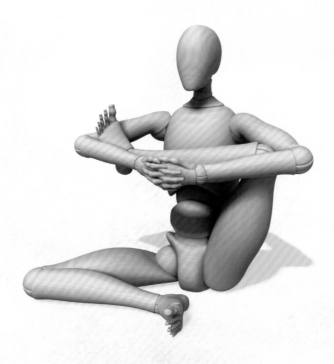

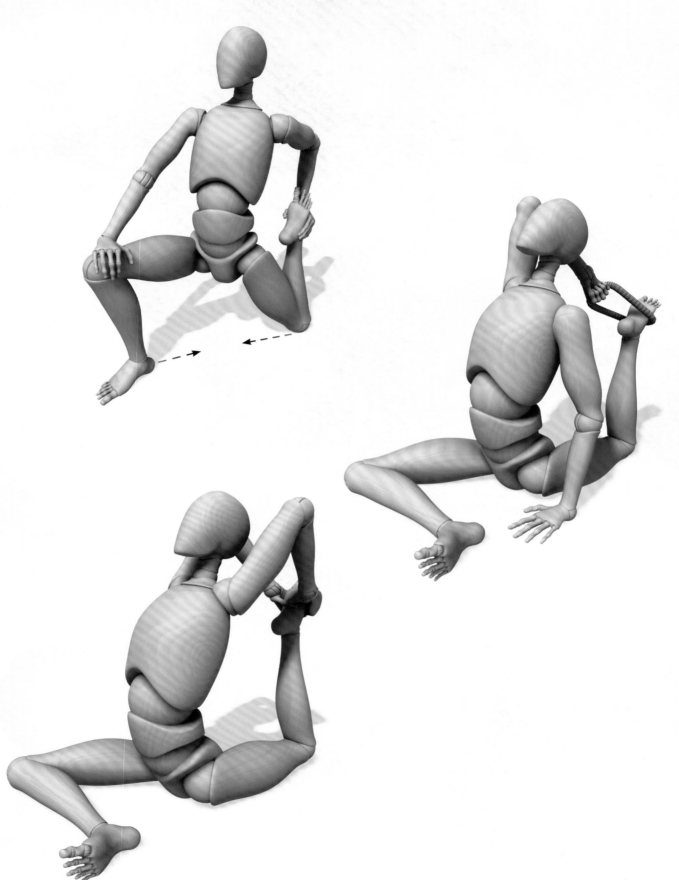

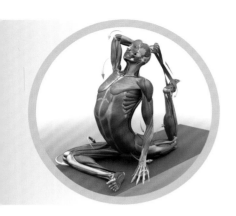

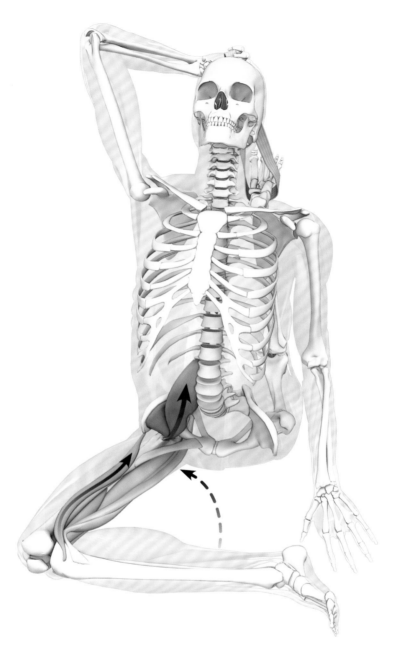

STEP 1 Contract the psoas and its synergists, the pectineus and adductors longus and brevis, to flex and externally rotate the thigh of the front leg. A cue for engaging the psoas is to press down on the knee while attempting to lift it off the ground. Observe how the psoas tilts the pelvis forward into anteversion and straightens the lower back. These movements work in rhythm with flexing and externally rotating the femur. Tilting the pelvis forward has the added benefit of releasing the iliofemoral ligament of the back hip. This ligament can limit extension of that hip and block deepening of the pose. Releasing it frees the back hip to extend further.

You can feel the sartorius running from the front of the pelvis to the inside of the knee. This muscle assists in flexing, abducting, and externally rotating the femur. Engage the hamstrings to flex the knee joint and use them to maintain it as a hinge.

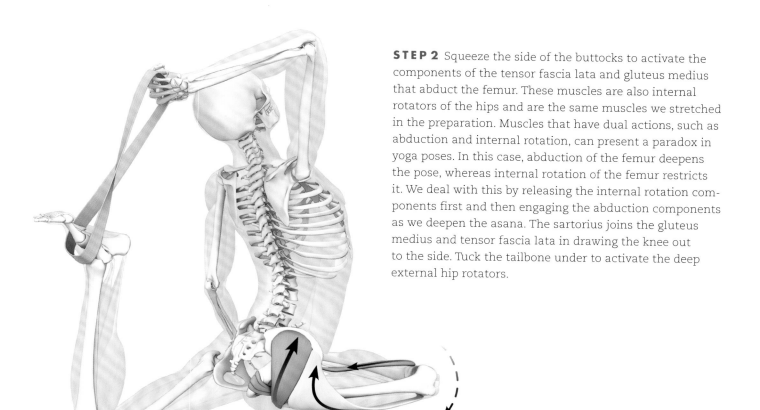

STEP 2 Squeeze the side of the buttocks to activate the components of the tensor fascia lata and gluteus medius that abduct the femur. These muscles are also internal rotators of the hips and are the same muscles we stretched in the preparation. Muscles that have dual actions, such as abduction and internal rotation, can present a paradox in yoga poses. In this case, abduction of the femur deepens the pose, whereas internal rotation of the femur restricts it. We deal with this by releasing the internal rotation components first and then engaging the abduction components as we deepen the asana. The sartorius joins the gluteus medius and tensor fascia lata in drawing the knee out to the side. Tuck the tailbone under to activate the deep external hip rotators.

▶ **STEP 3** The back hip extends, adducts, and internally rotates. Contract the gluteus maximus to extend the hip. Note that engaging this muscle also externally rotates the femur. We want to internally rotate it in Pigeon Pose. Do this by engaging the gluteus medius and tensor fascia lata. The cue for this is to press the back thigh and knee into the mat and attempt to drag it out to the side (abduct it). The mat will constrain the knee so that no abduction will actually occur; however, this engages the gluteus medius and tensor fascia lata and internally rotates the femur, as shown. The more posterior fibers of the gluteus medius also synergize the gluteus maximus in extending the hip. Contract the adductor magnus by drawing the knee towards the midline. Note how this improves hip extension.

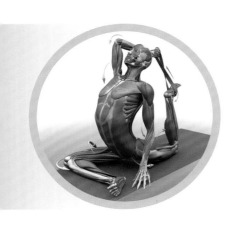

▶ **STEP 4** Expand the chest forward by arching the back; this activates the erector spinae and other deep extensor muscles of the spine, including the quadratus lumborum. Contract the lower portion of the trapezius to draw the shoulders away from the ears, and engage the rhomboids to bring the scapulae toward one another. This opens the chest like a pigeon. Improve this opening by contracting the pectoralis minor and serratus anterior muscles, as described in the Key Concepts.

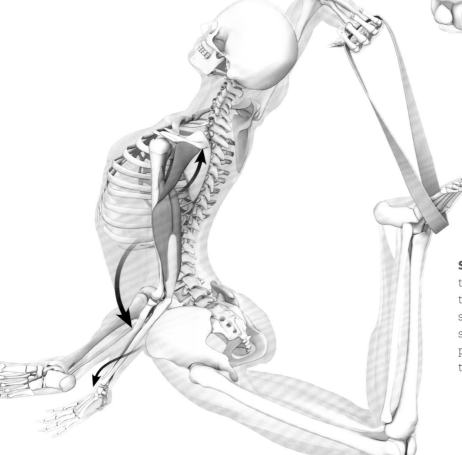

STEP 5 Use the hand on the floor to lift the chest. Push down into the mat to fix the hand by contracting the triceps and straightening the elbow. Then attempt to scrub backwards, activating the posterior portion of the deltoid. These actions lift the chest forward and up.

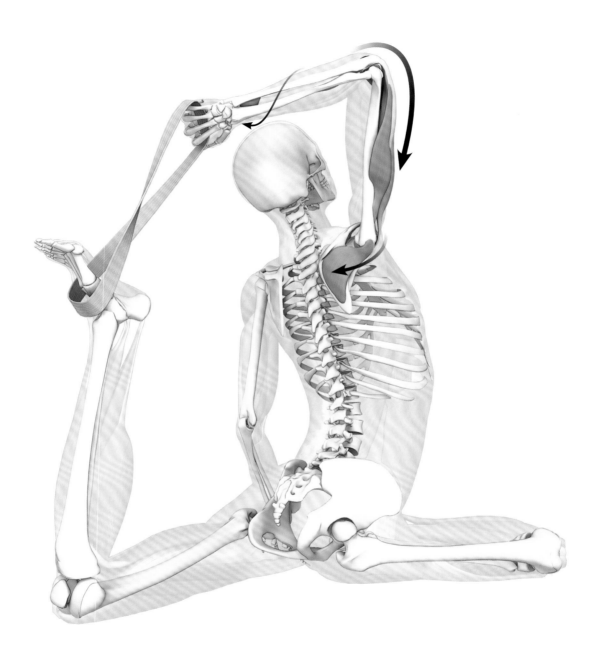

STEP 6 Use the upper hand to create a deeper extension of the back. Grasp the belt and pronate the forearm to rotate the palm to face upward as shown. This engages the pronator teres and quadratus muscles. Contract the triceps to attempt to straighten the elbow, and externally rotate the shoulders by engaging the infraspinatus and teres minor muscles. The force of these actions is transmitted to the chest, drawing it upward.

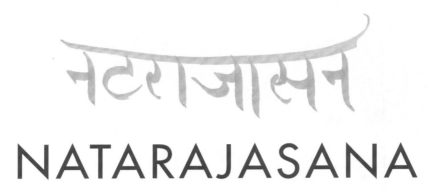

NATARAJASANA

DANCER POSE

DANCER POSE PRESENTS THE CHALLENGES OF COMBINING A BACKBEND WITH a one-legged balancing pose. Understanding these two distinct plot lines provides a starting point for achieving this advanced posture. As a general rule, it's best to separate out certain difficult aspects of a pose while mastering others. For example, distinguish the backbending story from the balancing act. Become proficient at each of these first and then combine the two.

Begin with the backbending component of the pose. The ability to deeply extend the hip and leg is a pre-requisite to Natarajasana. Accordingly, gain flexibility by stretching the psoas and its synergists, the pectineus, adductors longus and brevis, and sartorius. Use isolated stretches to achieve length in these muscles, and then apply this new flexibility to other backbending poses, such as Urdhva Dhanurasana and Ustrasana. Next, fine-tune your balance by practicing poses such as Vrksasana (Tree Pose) and Utthita Hasta Padangusthasana. Work toward Dancer by linking the upper hand and foot wth a belt, keeping the other hand on the wall to balance.

This demonstrates how to deconstruct a pose into its component parts, prepare those parts, use props, and finally reconstruct the pose into the classical asana. Remember that it's the journey that counts—each part of the process benefits you. Each part of the journey is yoga.

BASIC JOINT POSITIONS

- The standing-leg knee extends.
- The standing-leg hip flexes.
- The trunk extends.
- The held-leg hip extends.
- The held-leg knee flexes.
- The ankle plantar flexes.

- The shoulder of the arm that holds the foot flexes; its elbow flexes and forearm supinates.
- The free-arm shoulder flexes; its elbow extends and forearm pronates.

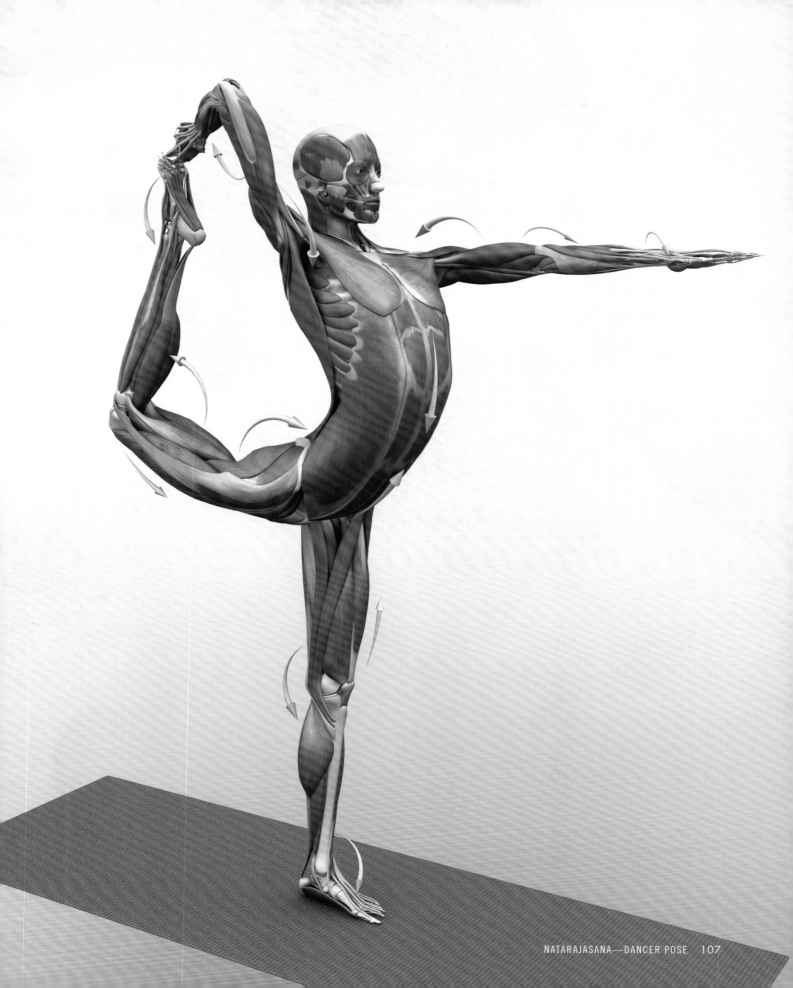

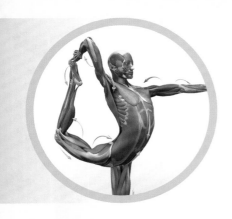

Natarajasana Preparation

Facilitated stretching is the most effective method for gaining length in muscles and is especially necessary in the quest to achieve such advanced poses as Natarajasana. You can apply facilitated stretching to lengthen the hip flexors with the psoas stretch shown here. Use a chair to open the shoulders. Add a facilitated component to this by intermittently pressing the elbows onto the seat of the chair; then take up the length gained by the relaxation response.

Once you have prepared the stretching muscles in this manner, you can begin working on the actual pose. Grasp the ankle while using the wall for support. In the beginning, this may be as far as you want to go. As your flexibility increases, lift the ankle behind you (with the arm extended back). This is one variation of the final pose. Another option is to flex the arm over the head (as in Urdhva Dhanurasana) and reach back to grasp the big toe. Use a belt to link to the foot at any time.

To come out of the pose, brace the body by contracting the quadriceps of the straight leg. Then bend the back knee and carefully exit. Take as long as is necessary to achieve this advanced posture—several months (or even years) if that's what it takes. Or stop along the way. Remember that consistency and slow progress is more important than overdoing it. Go step by step toward achieving your goal.

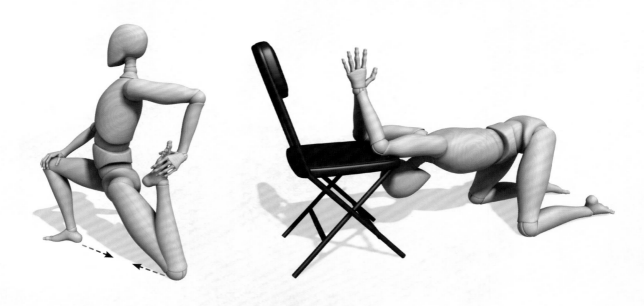

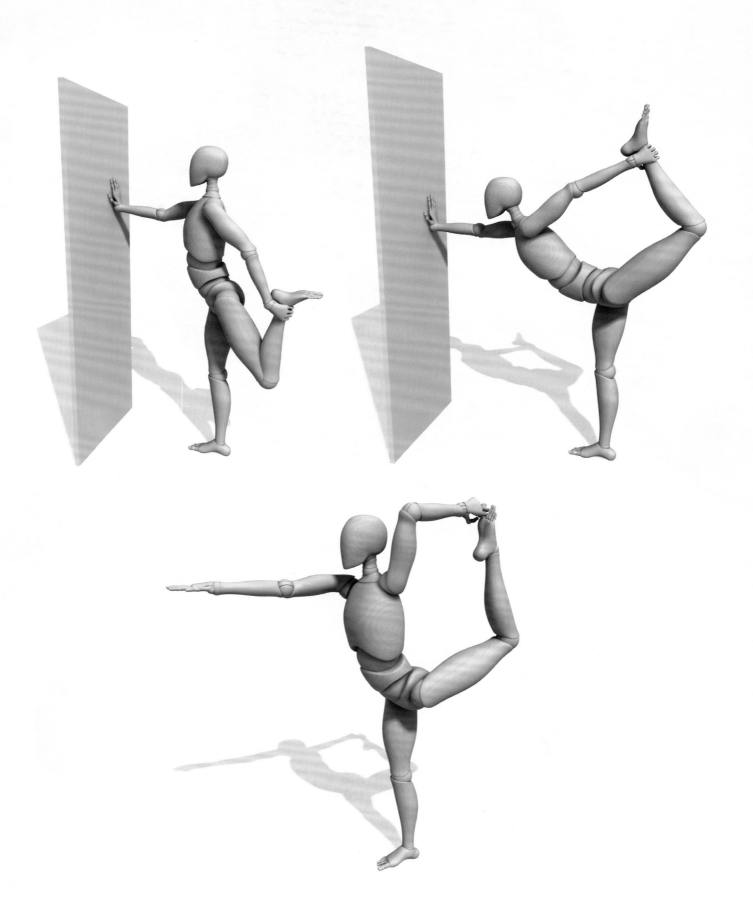

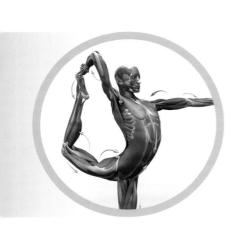

STEP 1 Several muscle groups are active in the standing leg. The hip abductors (the tensor fascia lata and gluteus medius) automatically engage when we stand on one leg. This tethers and balances the pelvis by pulling on the origins of these muscles at the iliac crest. If the adductors are weak or paralyzed, the pelvis sags over to the side of the leg that is in the air. This is known in medicine as the "Trendelenburg sign." Visualize these muscles at work to better stabilize the pose from the pelvic core.

The quadriceps contract to straighten the knee and the tensor fascia lata synergizes this action, in addition to stabilizing the knee joint from the outside. Press the ball of the foot into the mat to engage the peroneus longus and brevis. Then spread the weight across the sole by activating the tibialis posterior (this muscle everts the ankle). Use the toe flexors to refine your balance. Remember that primary stability originates from the pelvis. Refined stability is an interplay among the various muscles of the foot and ankle.

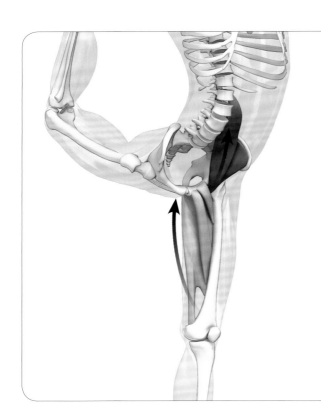

STEP 2 The psoas and adductor group engage to position the standing leg. Note how the psoas connects the lumbar spine to the femur, aiding to arch the back. This muscle also wraps over the front of the pelvis. Accordingly, contracting the psoas tilts the pelvis and trunk forward.

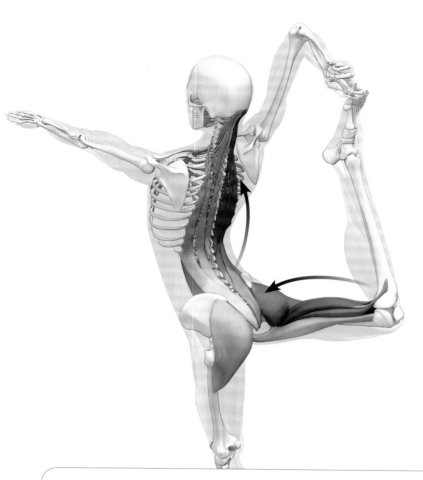

STEP 3 The hamstrings and gluteus maximus combine to lift the back leg. Squeeze the buttocks and tuck the tailbone during this phase. Later you will relax the hamstrings and engage their antagonists (the quadriceps) to deepen the arch. The knee will tend to drift out to the side as you lift the leg. Counter this by engaging the adductor magnus to draw the thigh toward the midline. This will also synergize the action of the gluteus maximus in extending the hip.

Arch the back by contracting the erector spinae and quadratus lumborum. Engage these muscles slightly more on the side of the lifted leg. The standing-leg gluteus maximus also contracts to assist you in balancing.

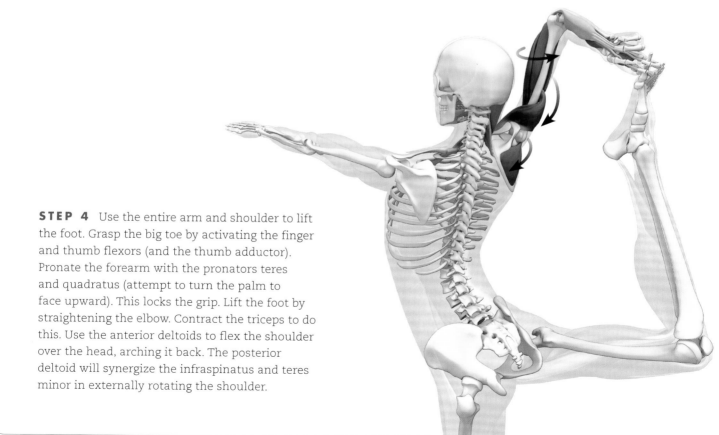

STEP 4 Use the entire arm and shoulder to lift the foot. Grasp the big toe by activating the finger and thumb flexors (and the thumb adductor). Pronate the forearm with the pronators teres and quadratus (attempt to turn the palm to face upward). This locks the grip. Lift the foot by straightening the elbow. Contract the triceps to do this. Use the anterior deltoids to flex the shoulder over the head, arching it back. The posterior deltoid will synergize the infraspinatus and teres minor in externally rotating the shoulder.

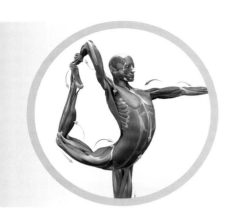

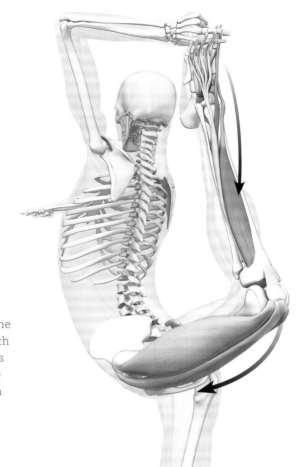

STEP 5 Attempt to dorsiflex the foot by contracting the tibialis anterior and toe extensors. The cue for this is to draw the top of the foot toward the shin. This further locks the grip on the big toe. Engage the quadriceps to deepen the arch of the back. Note how contracting these muscles straightens the knee and lifts the torso. Because these muscles also stretch in the pose, this is an eccentric contraction.

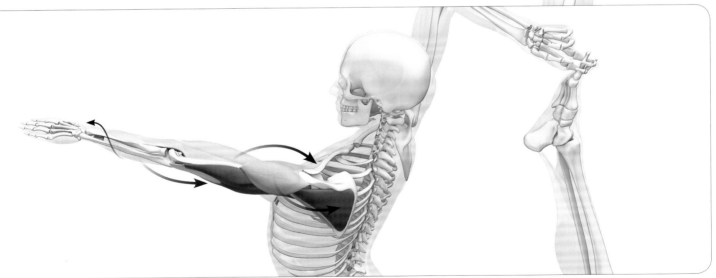

STEP 6 Activate the triceps to straighten the arm. Lift (forward flex) the shoulder with the anterior and lateral portions of the deltoid. Externally rotate the humerus by engaging the infraspinatus and teres minor; the posterior deltoid synergizes this action. Finally, create a coil down the arm by pronating the forearm using the pronators teres and quadratus. The cue for this is to turn the palm to face down. Moving the forearm in the opposite direction of the shoulders (which externally rotate) tightens the ligaments across the elbow and stabilizes the joint, creating a bandha.

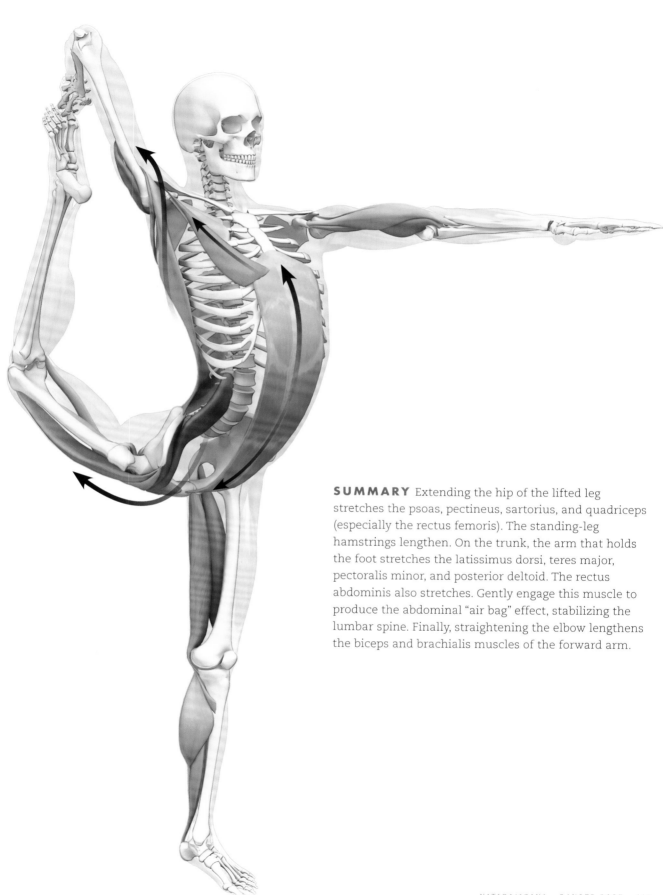

SUMMARY Extending the hip of the lifted leg stretches the psoas, pectineus, sartorius, and quadriceps (especially the rectus femoris). The standing-leg hamstrings lengthen. On the trunk, the arm that holds the foot stretches the latissimus dorsi, teres major, pectoralis minor, and posterior deltoid. The rectus abdominis also stretches. Gently engage this muscle to produce the abdominal "air bag" effect, stabilizing the lumbar spine. Finally, straightening the elbow lengthens the biceps and brachialis muscles of the forward arm.

TWISTS

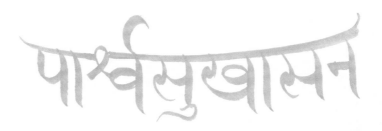

PARSVA SUKHASANA

EASY SEATED TWIST POSE

TWISTING POSES CONNECT THE UPPER AND LOWER APPENDICULAR SKELETONS (the arms and the legs) to turn the axial skeleton (the spine and torso). This lengthens the spinal rotator muscles that attach from one vertebra to another, as well as the erector spinae, quadratus lumborum, and abdominal musculature. It is important to understand how moving one part of the body affects another more distant part. This is a central tenet of yoga and is one factor that separates yoga from Western physical therapy. Most Western medical systems look at an isolated region of the body and develop exercises that focus on the structures within that region. Yoga looks at the entire body in a pose, and a pose within the practice, the practice integrated into life, and so on.

Note how bending the arm that is on the knee turns the trunk, which then turns the pelvis, affecting the legs. The legs and pelvis provide an anchoring counterforce by turning the lower body away from the chest and torso. The shoulder and pelvic girdles are connected by the vertebral column, which rotates to accommodate the twist. The form of Parsva Sukhasana illustrates how a variety of subplots or stories within the pose work together to affect the main theme—turning the upper body in one direction and the lower body in the other.

BASIC JOINT POSITIONS

- The hips flex, abduct, and externally rotate.
- The knees flex.
- The trunk extends and rotates.
- The shoulder on the side that holds the knee flexes; its elbow extends and forearm pronates.
- The back-arm shoulder extends; its elbow extends and forearm pronates.
- The cervical spine rotates.

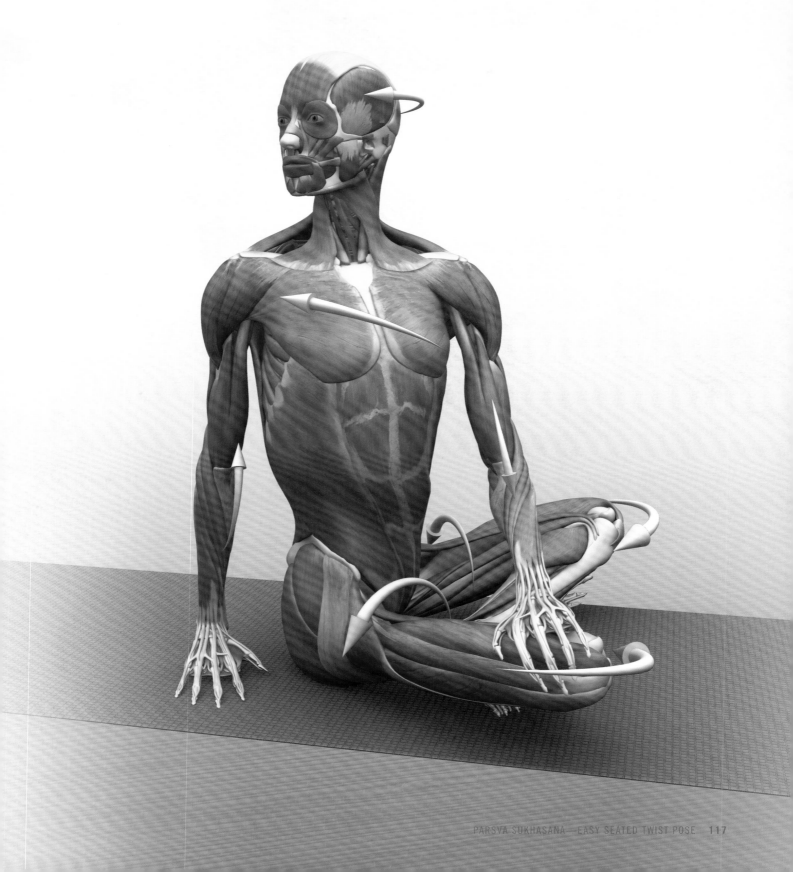

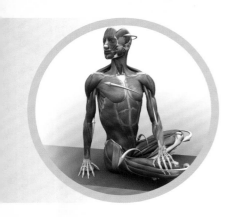

Parsva Sukhasana Preparation

The initial tendency in sitting cross-legged is for the back to slump, as shown here. An effective technique for drawing the spine to an erect and stable position is as follows: fix the hands on the knees and attempt to draw back by bending the elbows, as if you were pulling the knees toward you. The hands and knees won't move, but the chest will open forward and the spine will lift. This is the result of closed chain contraction of the latissimus dorsi. In this type of contraction, the insertion of the muscle remains fixed, because the arms don't actually move. Instead, the origin of the latissimus dorsi along the midline of the back is drawn forward, opening the chest.

Place one hand on the opposite knee and the other behind you on the floor. Press down into the floor to lift the chest. Bend the elbow of the hand that is on the knee to pull the torso into the twist. Attempt to drag the hand that is on the floor forward. That hand is now also fixed, and so the force generated by this action is transmuted into the twist, turning the upper body. Resist with the lower legs by abducting and externally rotating the thigh that you turn away from. This grounds the pelvis.

The variation of Parivrtta Parsvakonasana shown here can be used to create flexibility in the twist. Conversely, the seated twist can be used to prepare for the turning versions of standing poses. This illustrates the interrelatedness among the various categories of asanas.

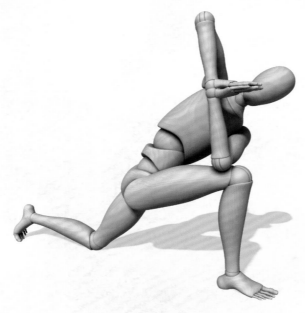

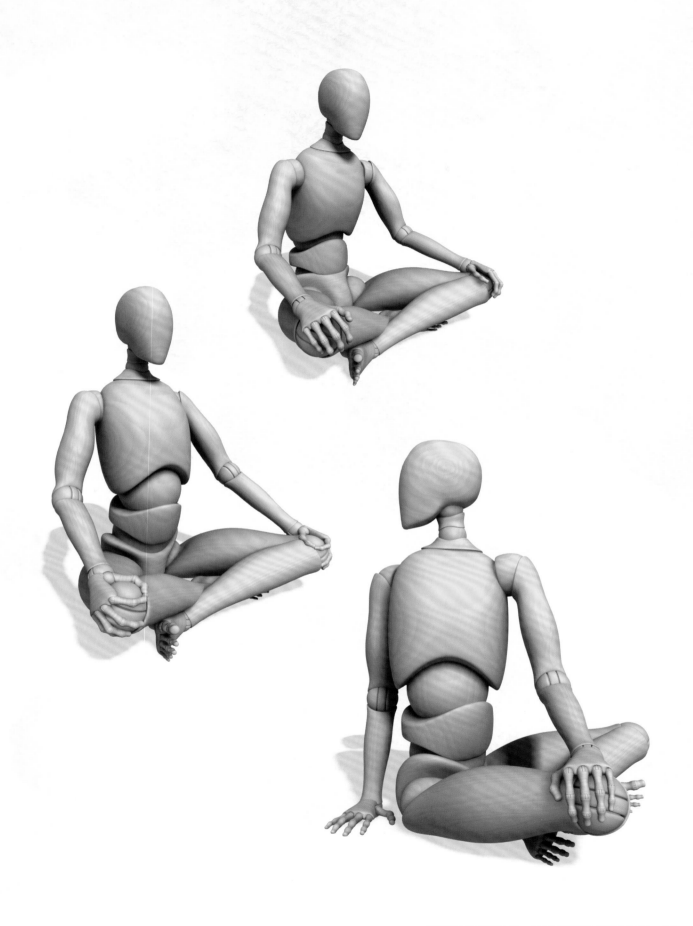

PARSVA SUKHASANA—EASY SEATED TWIST POSE   119

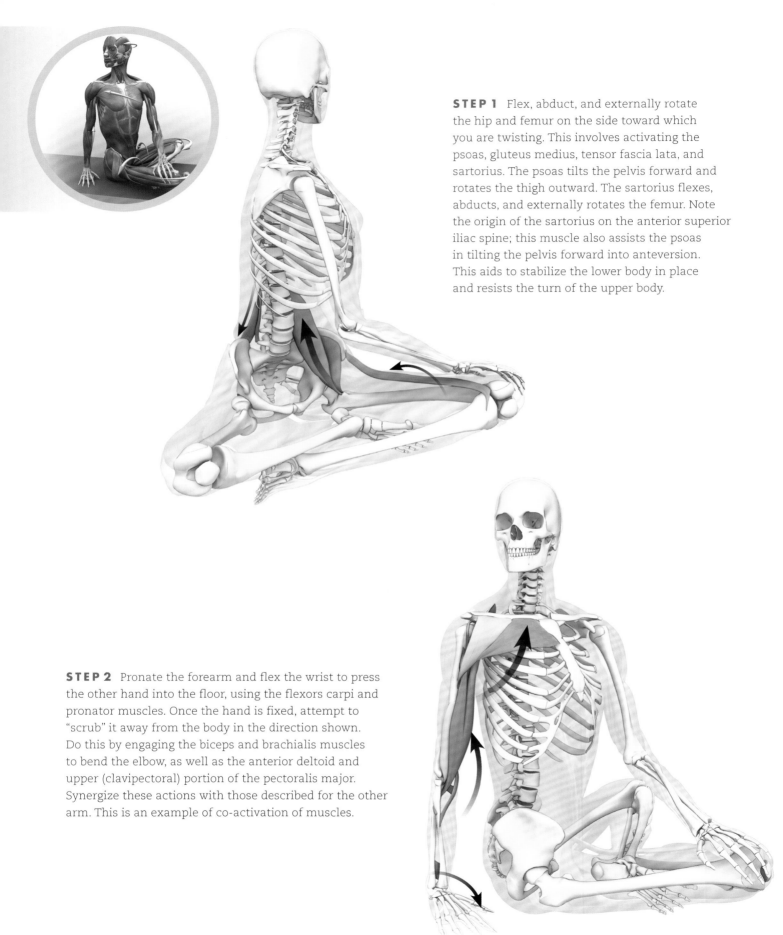

STEP 1 Flex, abduct, and externally rotate the hip and femur on the side toward which you are twisting. This involves activating the psoas, gluteus medius, tensor fascia lata, and sartorius. The psoas tilts the pelvis forward and rotates the thigh outward. The sartorius flexes, abducts, and externally rotates the femur. Note the origin of the sartorius on the anterior superior iliac spine; this muscle also assists the psoas in tilting the pelvis forward into anteversion. This aids to stabilize the lower body in place and resists the turn of the upper body.

STEP 2 Pronate the forearm and flex the wrist to press the other hand into the floor, using the flexors carpi and pronator muscles. Once the hand is fixed, attempt to "scrub" it away from the body in the direction shown. Do this by engaging the biceps and brachialis muscles to bend the elbow, as well as the anterior deltoid and upper (clavipectoral) portion of the pectoralis major. Synergize these actions with those described for the other arm. This is an example of co-activation of muscles.

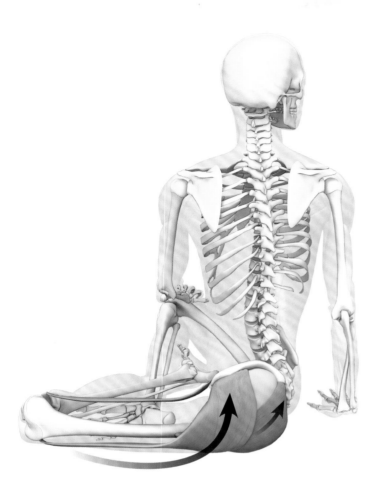

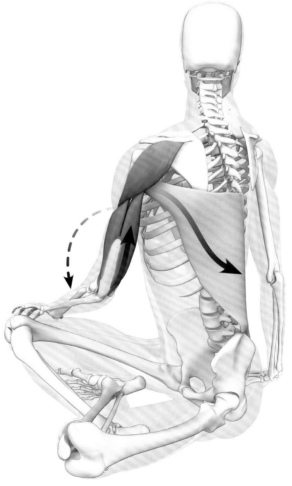

STEP 3 Engage the sartorius to flex, abduct, and externally rotate the hip and femur of the leg that is not held by the hand to turn the pelvis away from the upper body. Observe how this muscle feels like a cord running diagonally across the thigh. Squeeze the buttocks on this side to turn the thigh outward by externally rotating the hip. Activate the deep external rotators to tilt the pelvis back and down. This combines with the action of the psoas described in Step 3 to create a "wringing" effect across the sacroiliac ligaments, tightening them and stabilizing the pelvis. Draw the knee toward the floor to engage the abductors. The lumbar spine tends to bulge out on the opposite side as you turn. Counter this tendency by contracting the same-side quadratus lumborum.

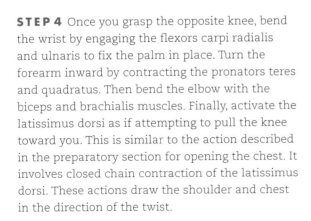

STEP 4 Once you grasp the opposite knee, bend the wrist by engaging the flexors carpi radialis and ulnaris to fix the palm in place. Turn the forearm inward by contracting the pronators teres and quadratus. Then bend the elbow with the biceps and brachialis muscles. Finally, activate the latissimus dorsi as if attempting to pull the knee toward you. This is similar to the action described in the preparatory section for opening the chest. It involves closed chain contraction of the latissimus dorsi. These actions draw the shoulder and chest in the direction of the twist.

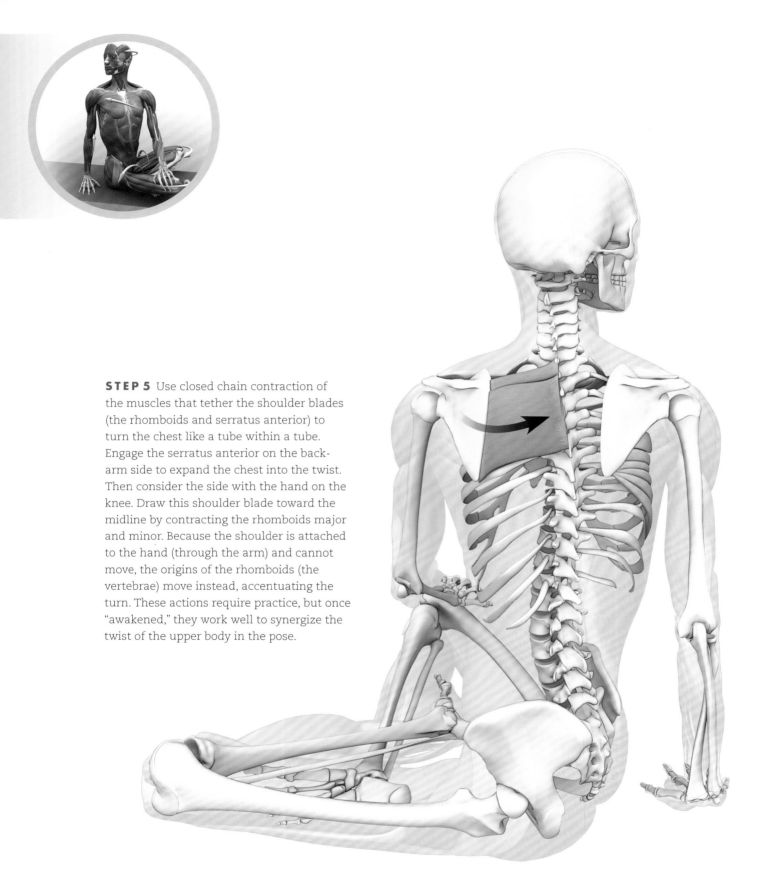

STEP 5 Use closed chain contraction of the muscles that tether the shoulder blades (the rhomboids and serratus anterior) to turn the chest like a tube within a tube. Engage the serratus anterior on the back-arm side to expand the chest into the twist. Then consider the side with the hand on the knee. Draw this shoulder blade toward the midline by contracting the rhomboids major and minor. Because the shoulder is attached to the hand (through the arm) and cannot move, the origins of the rhomboids (the vertebrae) move instead, accentuating the turn. These actions require practice, but once "awakened," they work well to synergize the twist of the upper body in the pose.

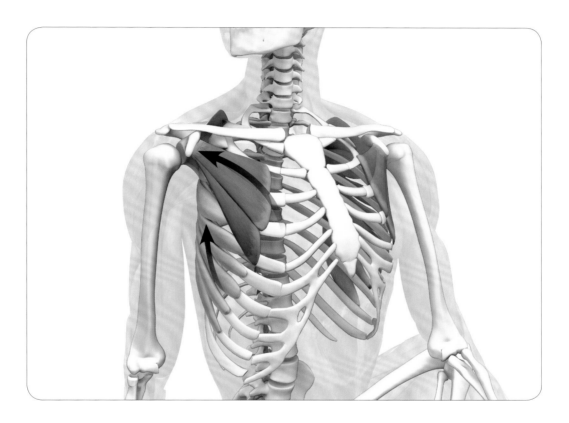

STEP 6 All twists tend to collapse the ribcage to some degree. This is because the thoracic spine has a limited capacity to rotate, being bound by the ribs. Use the accessory muscles of respiration to counteract this tendency. Begin by drawing the shoulder blades toward the midline and fixing them there. Then expand the chest by engaging the pectoralis minor and serratus anterior muscles.

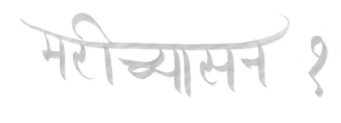

MARICHYASANA I

GREAT SAGE POSE

IN MARICHYASANA I WE ROTATE THE UPPER BODY AWAY FROM THE LOWER body. This is the main story of the pose. There are, however, a variety of smaller twists or subplots that contribute to the main story. For example, if we think of the lower body turning away from the upper body, then we can augment the twist of the lower body by turning the bent leg in a direction that synergizes the pose. To do this, we externally rotate the bent leg as a unit and internally rotate the straight leg. In this way, both lower extremities combine to turn the lower half of the body away from the upper. Similarly, we can rotate the shoulder on the bent-leg side down and toward the opposite leg while bringing the other shoulder up and back to turn the torso.

This combination of actions twists the shoulders and pelvis in opposite directions, moving the energy of nerve conduction upward through the susumna nadi in the torso. The key to this pose is seeking out all parts in the body that have the capacity to rotate and then combining them to deepen the twist.

BASIC JOINT POSITIONS

- The hips flex.
- The straight-leg knee extends.
- The held-leg knee flexes.
- The trunk flexes and rotates.

- The shoulders internally rotate and extend.
- The elbows extend and the forearms pronate.
- The held wrist extends.

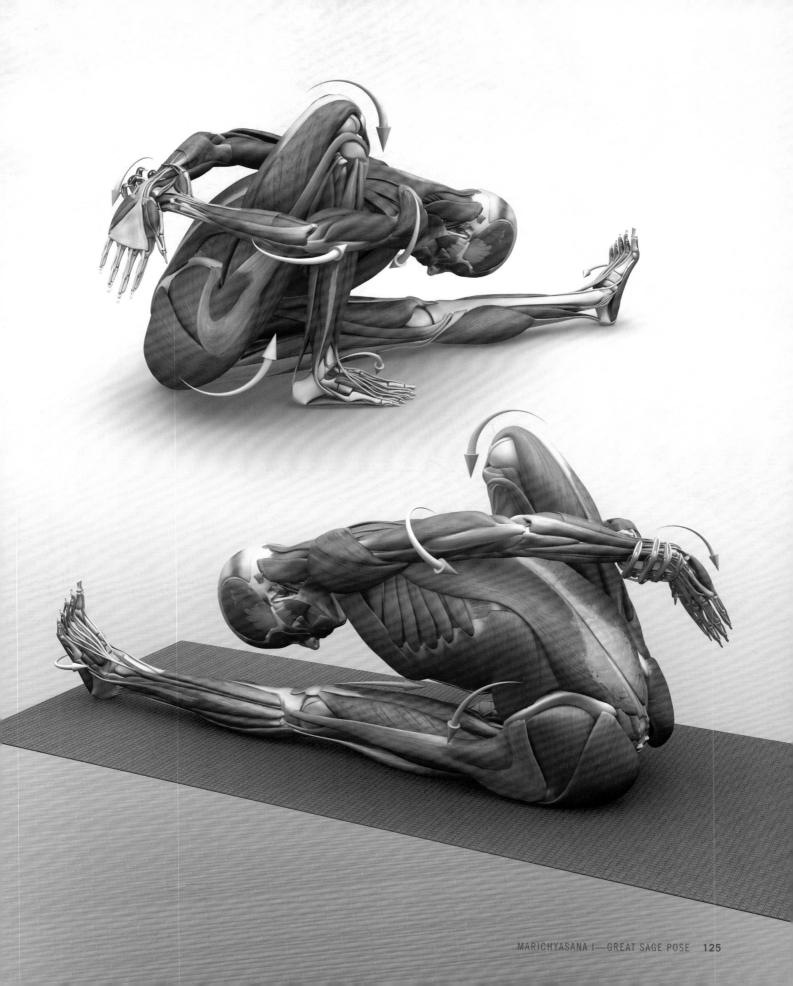

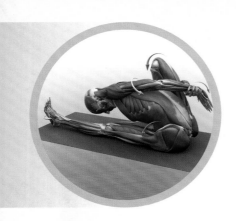

Marichyasana I Preparation

Begin in Dandasana. Take the general form of Marichyasana I by flexing the hip and bending the knee. Contract the hamstrings to squeeze the lower leg against the thigh and accentuate this bend. Activate the quadriceps of the straight leg to extend the knee. Bend forward and grasp the outstretched foot with the opposite hand; press the other hand into the floor beside the hip. Bend the elbow of the hand gripping the foot and attempt to straighten the other arm. Notice how this turns the body.

Next, reach behind the body and link the hands, either directly or with a belt. Initially, turn the shoulder on the bent-knee side forward while rolling the shoulder of the straight-leg side back. Flex the trunk over the straight leg. Once you are deep within the pose, draw the shoulders away from the ears. Ease out of the stretch by releasing the hands and turning the body toward the bent knee; sit up and straighten the leg, coming back to Dandasana.

To prepare for Marichyasana I, use poses such as the supine lunge illustrated here to gain flexibility in the bent-leg hip extensors.

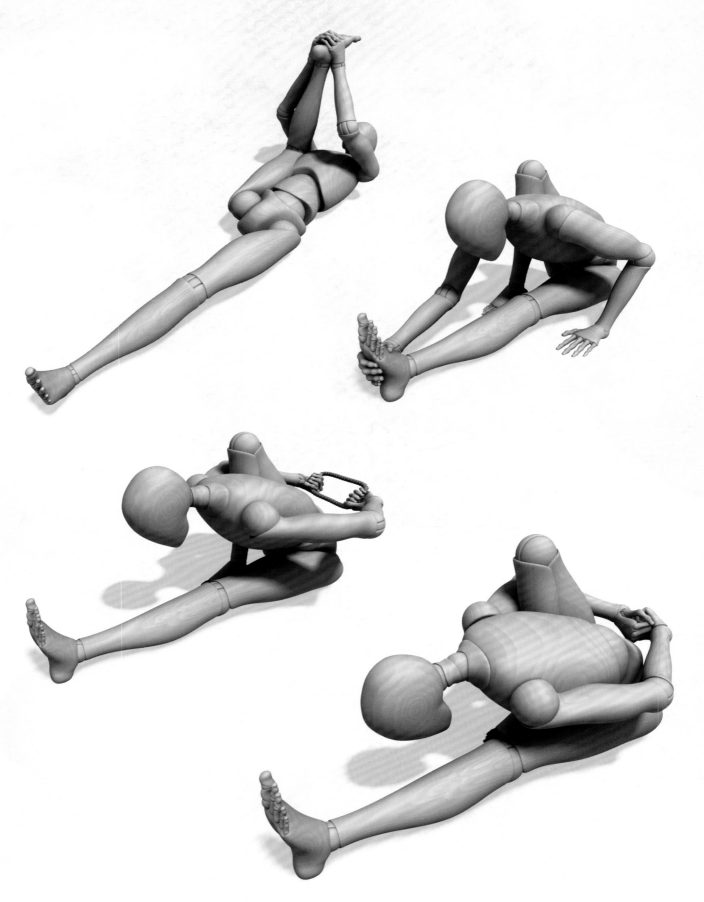

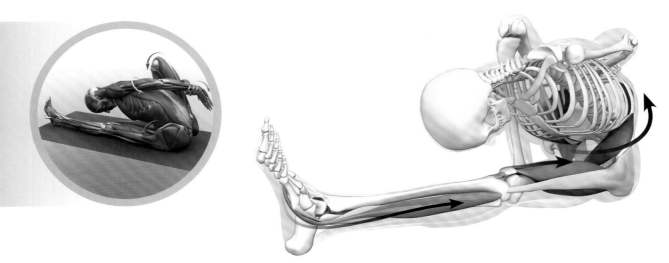

STEP 1 Extend the straight-leg knee by activating the quadriceps, and contract the peroneus longus and brevis muscles to turn the foot out slightly at the ankle and open the sole. Engage the tensor fascia lata. This synergizes the quadriceps in extending the knee and aids to flex the hip. The tensor fascia lata also contributes the important function of internally rotating the hip and femur of the straight leg. Bear in mind that the gluteus maximus stretches here because we are flexing forward. This creates a pull on the femur toward external rotation, turning the kneecap outward. The tensor fascia lata counteracts this, bringing the kneecap back to neutral.

STEP 2 Draw the trunk forward by contracting the abdominals. Both psoas muscles contribute to this action by flexing the hips. A cue for engaging the straight-leg psoas is to attempt to lift the leg off the floor; on the bent-leg side, squeeze the trunk against the leg. These actions tilt the pelvis forward and augment the stretch of the straight-leg hamstrings. Activate mula bandha to draw the coccyx forward and nutate the sacrum. This creates a counterbalance to the flexing trunk and stabilizes the pelvis.

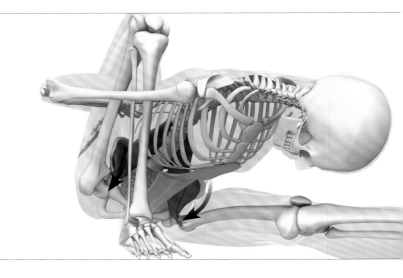

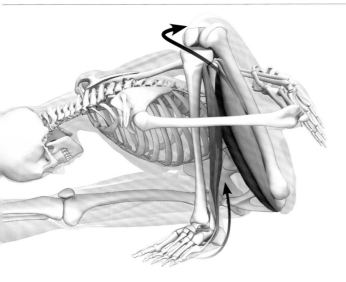

STEP 3 Contract the hamstrings to bend the knee. Remember that the inner-side hamstrings (the semimembranosus and semitendinosis) also internally rotate the tibia. Press the ball of the foot into the floor and gently rotate the foot inwards to engage these muscles. Note that when the lower leg is flexing against the upper, the two parts of the legs can be considered a single unit, like a log. This means that internally rotating the bent-leg tibia externally rotates the hip. Synergize this by tucking the tailbone under to engage the deep external rotators. This culminates in rolling the bent-leg side of the lower body away from the rotation of the upper body.

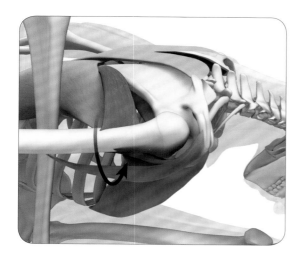

STEP 4 Both shoulders internally rotate, although the shoulder closer to the bent knee rotates inward slightly more to turn the upper body toward the straight leg. Get a feel for the muscles that produce this action before you actually do the pose. The cue for this is to put the hand behind the back at the level of the lumbar, and then lift it off. Use the other hand to feel how this activates the lower part of the pectoralis major and the deltoids. The latissimus dorsi, teres major, and subscapularis muscles work synergistically to internally rotate the shoulder.

STEP 5 To finish the pose, try to straighten the arms by contracting the triceps and draw the shoulders away from the neck by engaging the lower third of the trapezius. This levers the body forward. Use the posterior portion of the deltoids to lift the arms away from the back.

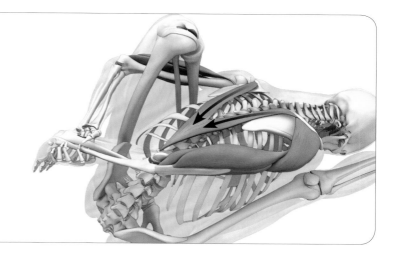

SUMMARY All of these actions culminate in a particular type of forward bend combined with a twist. In the lower body, the gluteus maximus of both legs and the hamstrings of the straight leg stretch. The back muscles, including the erector spinae, the spinal rotators, and the quadratus lumborum, all stretch. Internally rotating the shoulders stretches the infraspinatus and teres minor muscles, as well as parts of the deltoids.

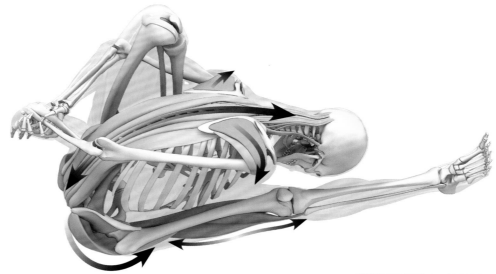

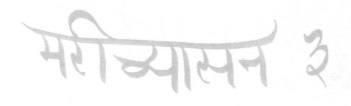

MARICHYASANA III
POSE DEDICATED TO THE SAGE MARICHI

IN THIS VERSION OF MARICHYASANA, WE TURN THE UPPER BODY AWAY FROM the straight leg and toward the flexing knee. Similarly, the lower body, from the pelvis down through the legs, turns away from the upper body. The twisting trunk and vertebral column connect the shoulders and hips. Each region of the body forms a subplot that contributes to the main story of the pose. For example, look how the upper and lower extremities connect where the upper arm wraps over the bent knee. This point forms a focus of leverage with different variations, depending on the way the arm and the leg are used. For example, fix the knee in place and then press against it with the arm to turn the body. Then brace the arm and push against it with the side of the leg. Note the different effects of these two actions. Finally, press the arm and leg equally against each other. How is your experience of the pose different in each variation? Work your way into the shoulders. Note that the rotator cuff (the deep muscles of the shoulder) can subtly augment the twist. The more superficial muscles, such as the deltoids and latissimus dorsi, also have rotational components, depending on the angles of the fibers. Then look at the bent leg. There are muscles with rotational actions from the foot to the hip; any of these can be engaged to augment the twist to varying degrees. Each forms a chapter in the story of the pose. The breath provides the soundtrack.

BASIC JOINT POSITIONS

- The hips flex.
- The straight-leg knee extends.
- The held-leg knee flexes.
- The trunk rotates.

- The shoulders internally rotate and extend.
- The elbows extend and the forearms pronate.
- The held wrist extends.

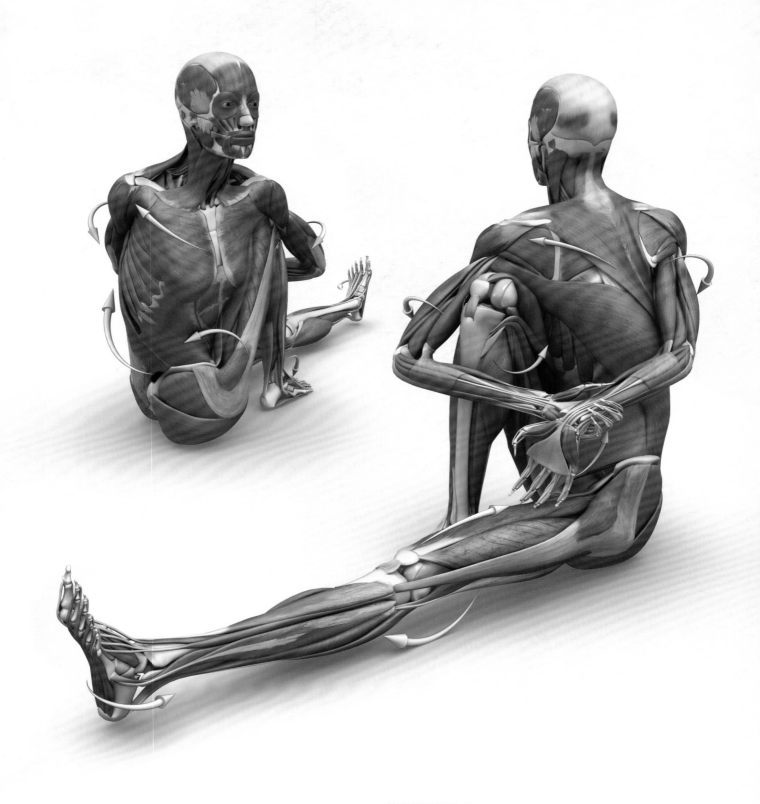

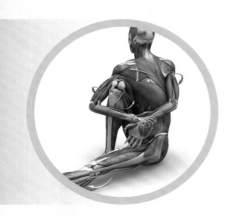

Marichyasana III Preparation

Reach around the knee and bend the elbow to draw the torso toward the thigh. Squeeze the knee into the chest. Then push the side of the leg into the hand and feel how this aids to turn the body. Press the other hand into the floor a few inches behind the sacrum, and straighten the elbow to lift the chest. Then attempt to scrub forward with the hand to augment the twist.

As you become more flexible, place the outer elbow against the knee. Then fix the knee and thigh in place as a stationary object and press the elbow against the side of the leg to turn the body. Vary this by fixing the elbow as a stationary object and pressing the knee into the back of the elbow. Finally, press the knee and the elbow equally into each other. Observe the different effects of these actions. Next, rotate the forward arm internally and reach the hand around the knee. Similarly, roll the back shoulder inward and reach the arm behind the back. Link the hands with a belt and pull with the hand that is wrapped around the knee to draw the upper body deeper into the twist. Eventually connect the hands, first by inter-locking the fingers and then by grasping the wrist, as illustrated here. Extend the wrist of the back arm to lock the grip.

Don't forget the storyline of the straight leg. As you twist further from the upper body, the straight leg will tend to rotate internally. Balance this by engaging the buttocks to press the back of the leg into the floor, and then externally rotate the thigh to bring the kneecap to face straight upwards.

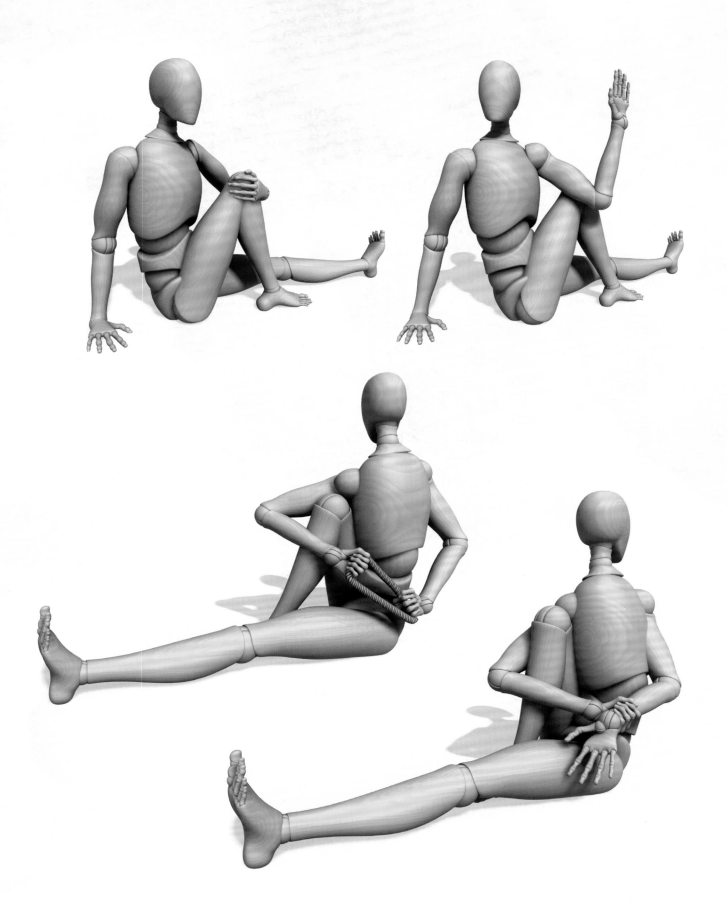

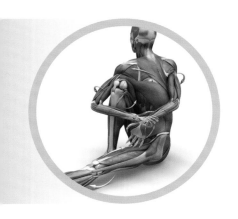

STEP 1 Flex the hip by activating the psoas and its synergists. Note the rhythmic action of the femur flexing and the pelvis tilting forward simultaneously. Contract the hamstrings to flex the knee. Remember that the knee has some capacity to rotate and thus contributes to the twist. Engage the outer hamstrings—the biceps femoris—to create this movement. The cue for this is to plant the ball of the foot into the mat and gently attempt to turn the foot in external rotation (as illustrated). With the knee bent, the thigh and lower leg move as a unit. This means that external rotation of the tibia internally rotates the hip. This action contributes to turning the lower body away from the upper body, deepening the twist.

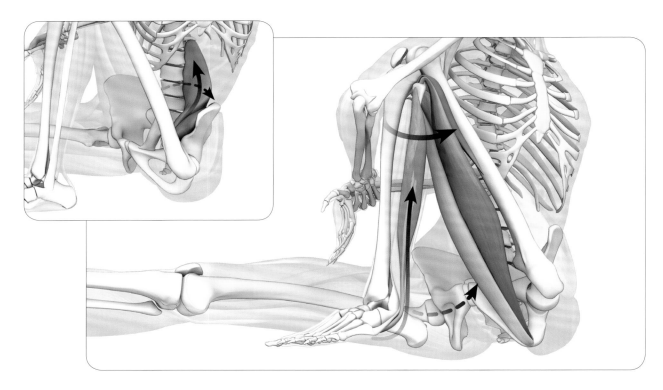

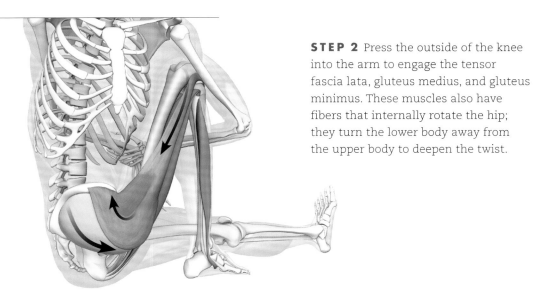

STEP 2 Press the outside of the knee into the arm to engage the tensor fascia lata, gluteus medius, and gluteus minimus. These muscles also have fibers that internally rotate the hip; they turn the lower body away from the upper body to deepen the twist.

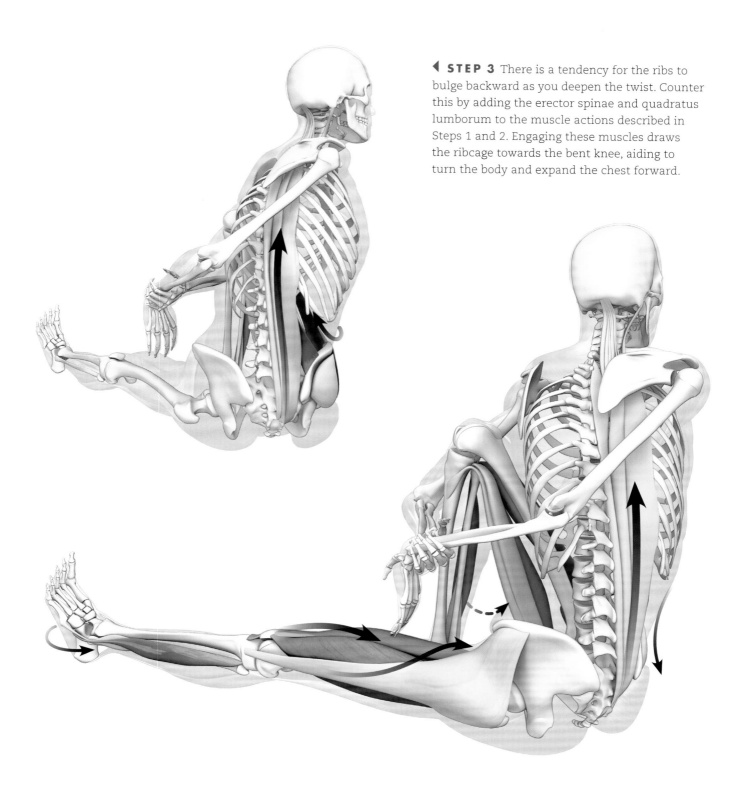

STEP 3 There is a tendency for the ribs to bulge backward as you deepen the twist. Counter this by adding the erector spinae and quadratus lumborum to the muscle actions described in Steps 1 and 2. Engaging these muscles draws the ribcage towards the bent knee, aiding to turn the body and expand the chest forward.

STEP 4 Activate the quadriceps to extend the straight-leg knee. The upper body will tend to draw this leg into some degree of internal rotation. We want to rotate it away from the upper body, but only to the point where the kneecap faces up (not more to one side or the other). Balance internal and external rotation of the thigh.

Engage the gluteus maximus by pressing the entire back of the leg into the floor. Tuck the tailbone under to activate the deep external rotators. These actions will turn the leg slightly outward and bring the kneecap to face straight up. Offset this by engaging the tensor fascia lata and gluteus medius to stabilize the thigh.

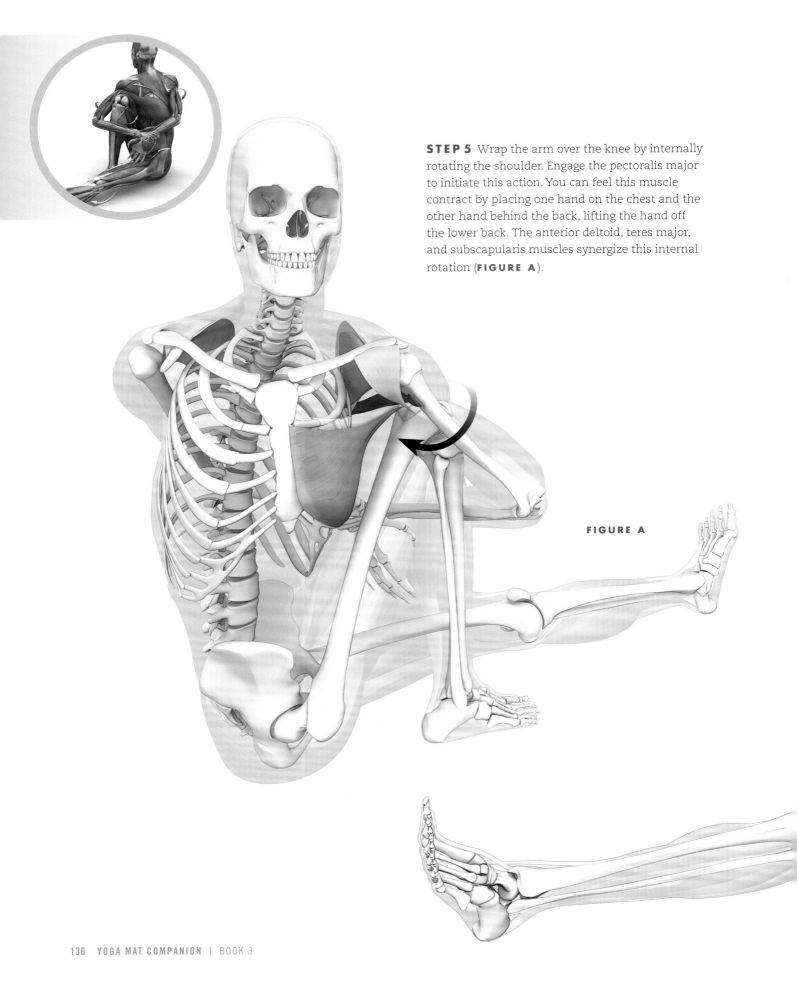

STEP 5 Wrap the arm over the knee by internally rotating the shoulder. Engage the pectoralis major to initiate this action. You can feel this muscle contract by placing one hand on the chest and the other hand behind the back, lifting the hand off the lower back. The anterior deltoid, teres major, and subscapularis muscles synergize this internal rotation (**FIGURE A**).

FIGURE A

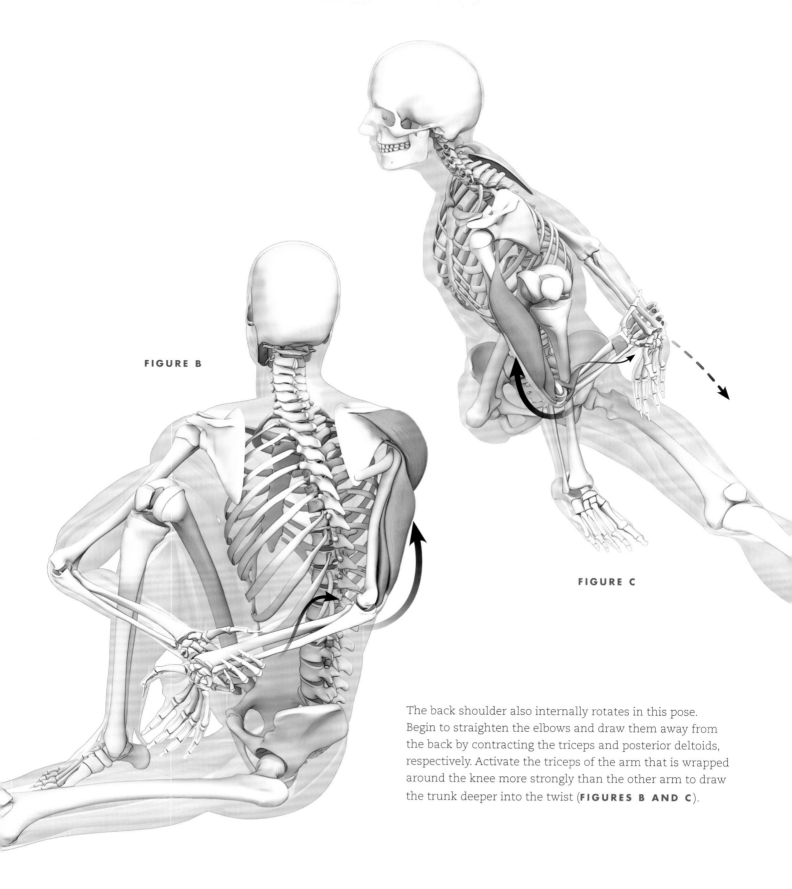

FIGURE C

The back shoulder also internally rotates in this pose. Begin to straighten the elbows and draw them away from the back by contracting the triceps and posterior deltoids, respectively. Activate the triceps of the arm that is wrapped around the knee more strongly than the other arm to draw the trunk deeper into the twist (**FIGURES B AND C**).

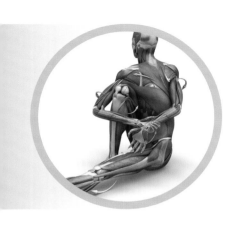

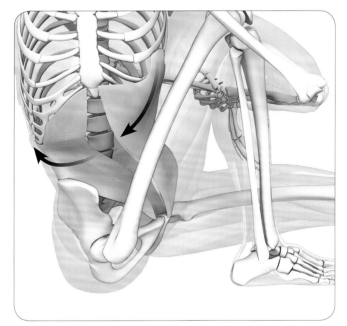

STEP 6 Engage the rhomboids to draw the back-arm shoulder blade towards the spine. Activate the serratus anterior to abduct the front-arm shoulder blade away from the midline (as if pushing an object away from you). These two actions synergize to turn the thorax (the chest) from the shoulders.

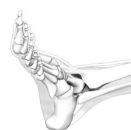

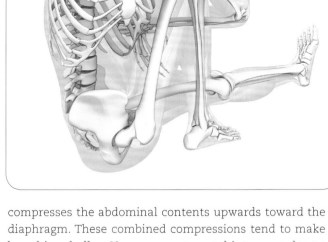

STEP 7 Rotate the forward shoulder toward the knee. This engages the forward-side internal oblique abdominals and the back-side external oblique abdominals. You can isolate these muscles by flexing the trunk forward toward the opposite knee. Turning the thorax contorts the ribcage and contracting the abdominal muscles compresses the abdominal contents upwards toward the diaphragm. These combined compressions tend to make breathing shallow. You can counteract this to some degree using the accessory muscles of breathing, especially the pectoralis minor and serratus anterior, to actively expand the ribcage.

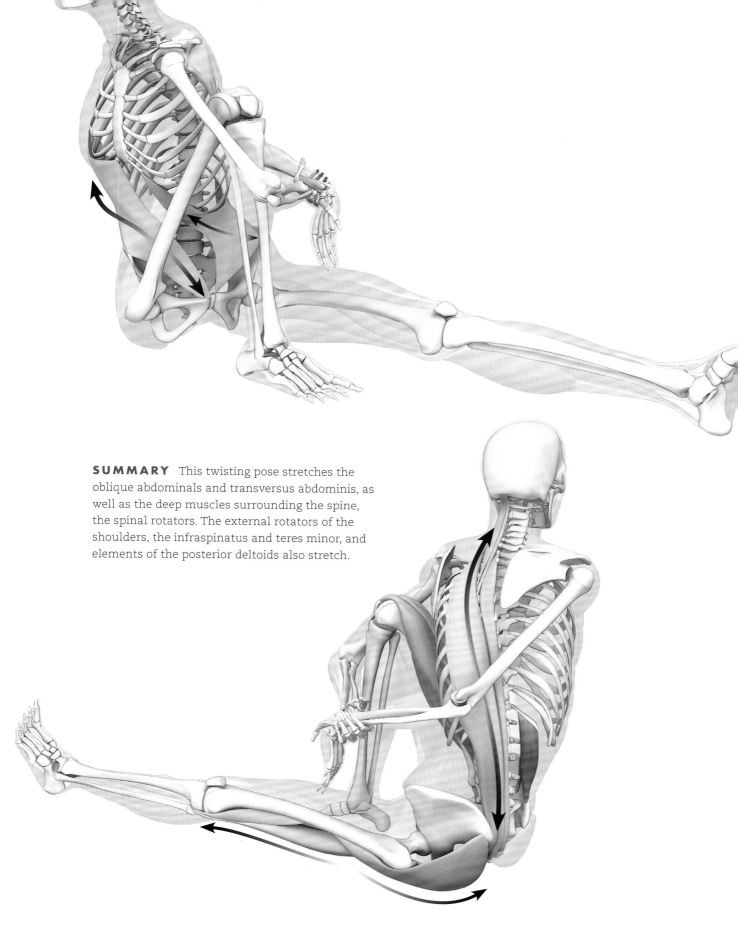

SUMMARY This twisting pose stretches the oblique abdominals and transversus abdominis, as well as the deep muscles surrounding the spine, the spinal rotators. The external rotators of the shoulders, the infraspinatus and teres minor, and elements of the posterior deltoids also stretch.

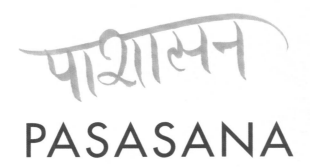

PASASANA

NOOSE POSE

EVERY POSE TELLS A STORY, AND EVERY STORY IS COMPRISED OF SUBPLOTS. BREAK Pasasana down into its component parts—the subplots of the main story. Then reconstruct these parts into the whole. See how each subplot contributes to the final pose. Yoga reveals the interrelationships between all parts of the body. This is one characteristic that distinguishes yoga from practices such as Western physical therapy, which tend to focus on specific regions (such as a painful shoulder or knee). Yoga looks at the whole. Nevertheless, we can learn from focusing on individual parts of a pose and then integrate this knowledge into the final posture. In Pasasana, for example, there are several specific actions that take place.

First look at the lower legs. The calf muscles stretch from dorsiflexing the feet and ankles. This stretch differs somewhat from that in Dog Pose. In the latter, the calves lengthen more in the region of the knees. Here the stretch is concentrated in the distal part of the muscle, where it blends into the Achilles tendon, which attaches to the heel. Actively dorsiflexing the ankle joint engages the tibialis anterior muscle at the front of the lower leg. At the same time, this signals the gastrocnemius and soleus muscles—antagonists of the tibialis anterior—to relax via reciprocal inhibition.

Next, look at the pelvis and hips. The hip that you twist toward flexes relatively more than the other hip. This leads to the knees being uneven. Balance this by extending the forward-leg hip (with the gluteus maximus) and flexing the back-leg hip (with the psoas). Note how this brings the knees even with each other. Lock this position by squeezing the knees together (with the adductor group). This creates a bandha in the pelvis, stabilizing the pose.

Finally, look at the shoulder girdle. Use the muscles of the shoulders and arms to gently leverage and rotate the upper body in the opposite direction of the lower, stretching the muscles of the trunk and back.

BASIC JOINT POSITIONS

- The hips flex and adduct.
- The knees flex.
- The ankles dorsiflex.
- The trunk flexes and rotates.

- The shoulders internally rotate and extend.
- The elbows extend and the forearms pronate.
- The held wrist extends.

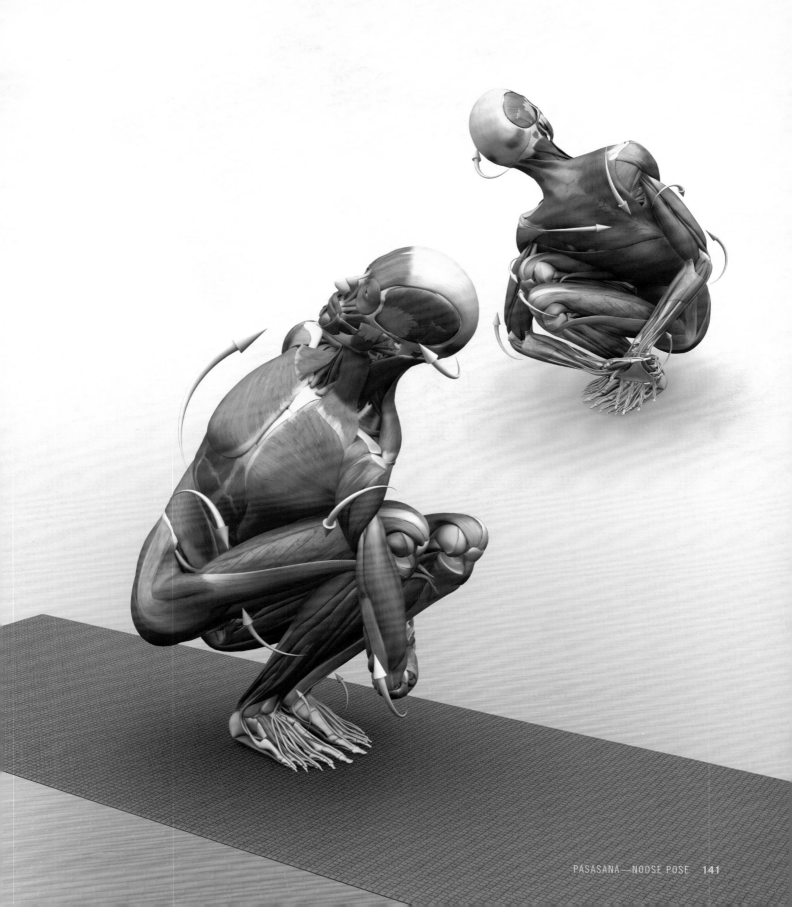

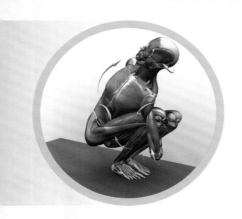

Pasasana Preparation

Use Downward Facing Dog Pose to stretch the calf muscles as a warm-up. Although the stretch of Downward Dog has a slightly different focus than Pasasana, it is still useful to gain length in the gastrocnemius and soleus muscles at the backs of the lower legs. Place the heels on a block in the beginning to aid in balance and to compensate for tightness in the calves. Actively engage the muscles at the fronts of the lower legs to bring the heels toward the floor (through dorsiflexion of the ankles).

Prepare the arms for internal rotation with reverse namasté (Paschima Namaskarasana) or Gomukhasana. Practice Marichyasana III to prepare the torso for the twist. If you can't link the arms behind the back, use a belt. Alternatively, try the chair twist shown here. Work toward placing the heels and soles of the feet onto the mat. Then brace the abdominals and carefully release the pose. You will see that the knees are uneven when you go into the twist. Follow the steps outlined in the muscles section to balance this and at the same time create a bandha.

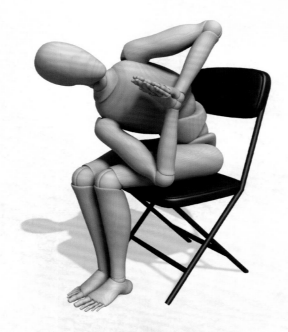

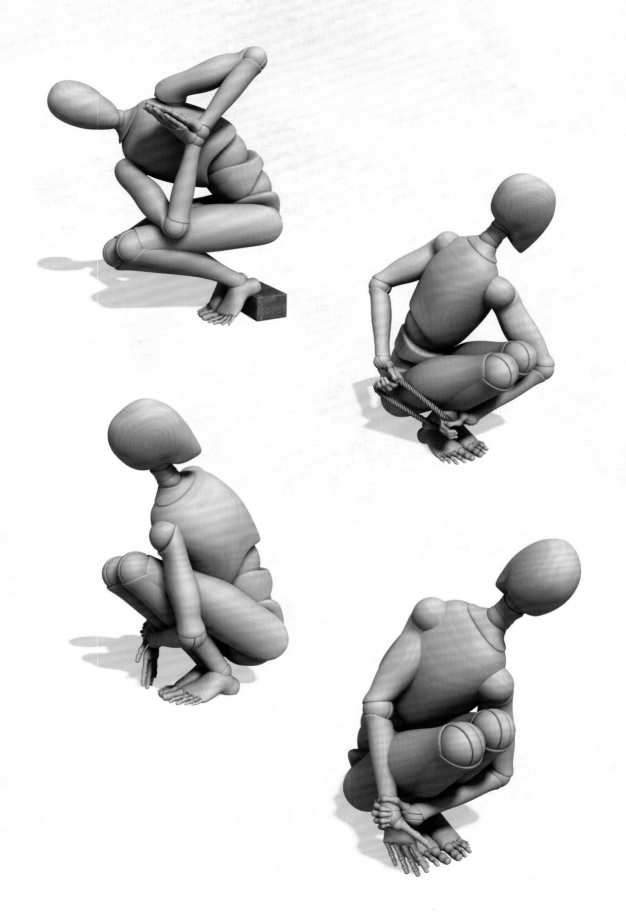

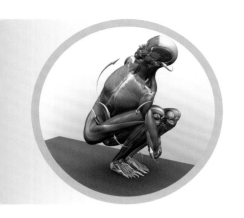

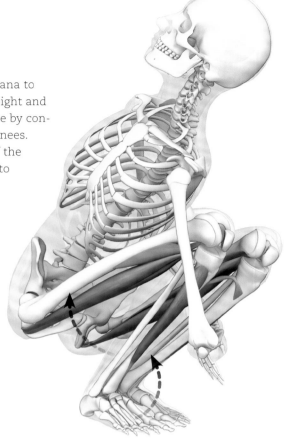

STEP 1 There is a tendency in Pasasana to flex the knees using only the body weight and gravity. Instead, make it an active pose by contracting the hamstrings to bend the knees. This produces reciprocal inhibition of the quadriceps, allowing them to relax into the stretch.

Dorsiflex the ankles to lower the heels. Do this by drawing the tops of the feet toward the fronts of the shins. This activates the tibialis anterior muscles at the fronts of the lower legs, at the same time signalling the gastrocnemius and soleus muscles to relax (reciprocal inhibition).

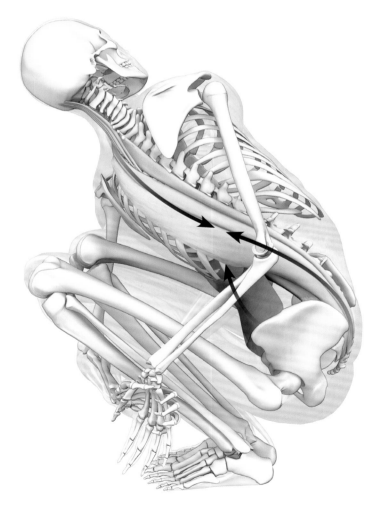

STEP 2 Laterally flex and turn the torso by engaging the lower-side oblique abdominals. Add to this lateral flexion by contracting the erector spinae and quadratus lumborum. The cue for this is to gently arch the back.

STEP 3 The knees will tend to be uneven due to the turned pelvis. Work toward bringing them together. Note that the hip you are turning toward is flexing more than the other hip. Balance this with extension by contracting the gluteus maximus (squeezing the buttocks) on this side. The other hip contributes to the unevenness because it is more extended. Address this by engaging the psoas (the main hip flexor) to bring the knees in line with each other. A cue for engaging this muscle is to squeeze the thigh upward against the torso. Co-activating these two muscles creates a "wringing" effect across the pelvis and tightens the sacroiliac ligaments (ligamentotaxis). The result is a bandha that stabilizes the pose.

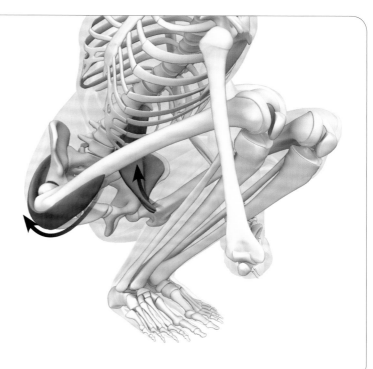

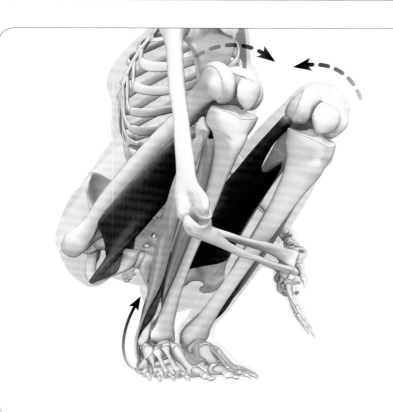

STEP 4 Once you have brought the knees in line with each other by engaging the muscles described in Step 3, lock them in place by contracting the adductor group on the insides of the thighs to squeeze the knees together. Then press the balls of the feet into the mat by activating the peroneus longus and brevis muscles at the sides of the lower legs. Balance this action by contracting the tibialis posterior to slightly invert the ankles and lift the arches of the feet. This aids to distribute the weight evenly across the soles.

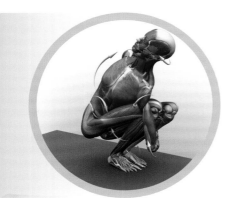

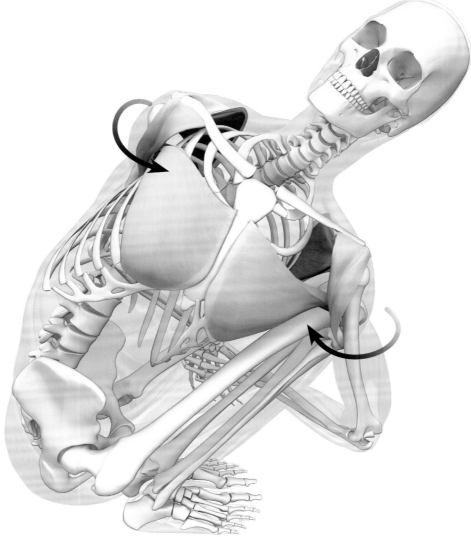

STEP 5 Engage the pectoralis major, anterior deltoids, and subscapularis muscles to internally rotate the shoulders. A cue for this is to imagine lifting the hands off the lower back.

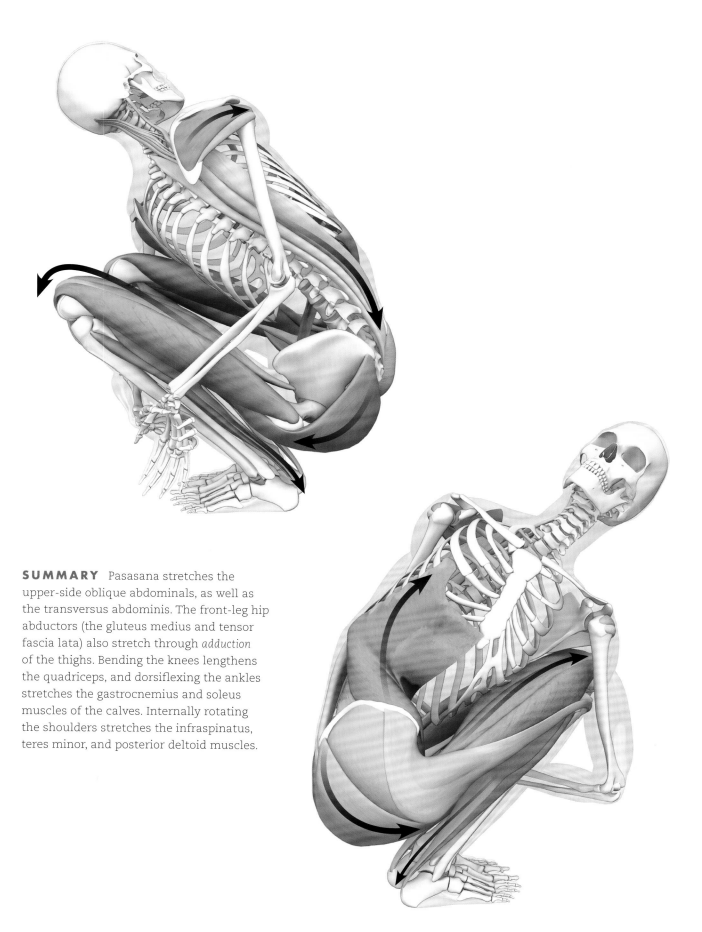

SUMMARY Pasasana stretches the upper-side oblique abdominals, as well as the transversus abdominis. The front-leg hip abductors (the gluteus medius and tensor fascia lata) also stretch through *adduction* of the thighs. Bending the knees lengthens the quadriceps, and dorsiflexing the ankles stretches the gastrocnemius and soleus muscles of the calves. Internally rotating the shoulders stretches the infraspinatus, teres minor, and posterior deltoid muscles.

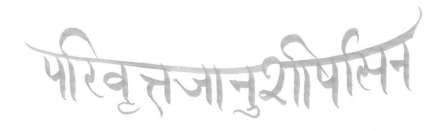

PARIVRTTA JANU SIRSASANA

REVOLVED HEAD-TO-KNEE POSE

SOME OF THE MOST PROFOUND EXPERIENCES IN YOGA OCCUR VIA MILLIMETERS of movement in just the right area. Seek out these experiences by finding interactivity between different parts of the body within your poses. For example, in Parivrtta Janu Sirsasana, observe how the back of the lower arm and elbow interact with the inside of the straight leg. How does this affect turning the torso? Note that pressing the back of the arm against the inner knee levers the chest to face upward. Bending the elbows flexes the torso further over the straight leg. Then look at the bent leg. If you externally rotate and abduct the thigh further back, the stretch of the upper-side trunk is increased.

Triangulate the focal points in the pose, and then activate the muscle groups to shine a light on the area of interest. For example, in Parivrtta Janu Sirsasana, contracting the shoulder flexors and bending the elbow while turning the back leg and anchoring the pelvis locates a focal point in the region of the upper-side oblique abdominals. Once you localize the muscles that are stretching, use the spinal cord reflexes to relax them. In this pose, the muscles of the shoulders that are deepening the stretch are not direct antagonists of the abdominals, so they don't produce reciprocal inhibition of these muscles. To create this effect, engage the lower-side abdominals—the direct antagonists—to relax the upper side. Then re-engage the muscles of the arms and legs to deepen the pose. This is one example of interactivity within a posture.

There are many such subplots in any asana. This technique of triangulation combines various subplots to highlight a region or group of muscles within a pose and then uses physiological reflexes to gain length in those muscles and space in the joints.

BASIC JOINT POSITIONS

- The bent-leg hip flexes, abducts, and externally rotates.
- The knee of the same leg flexes.
- The straight-leg hip flexes and externally rotates.
- The knee of the same leg extends.

- The trunk flexes and rotates.
- The shoulders abduct and flex.
- The elbows flex.
- The forearms supinate.
- The wrists flex.

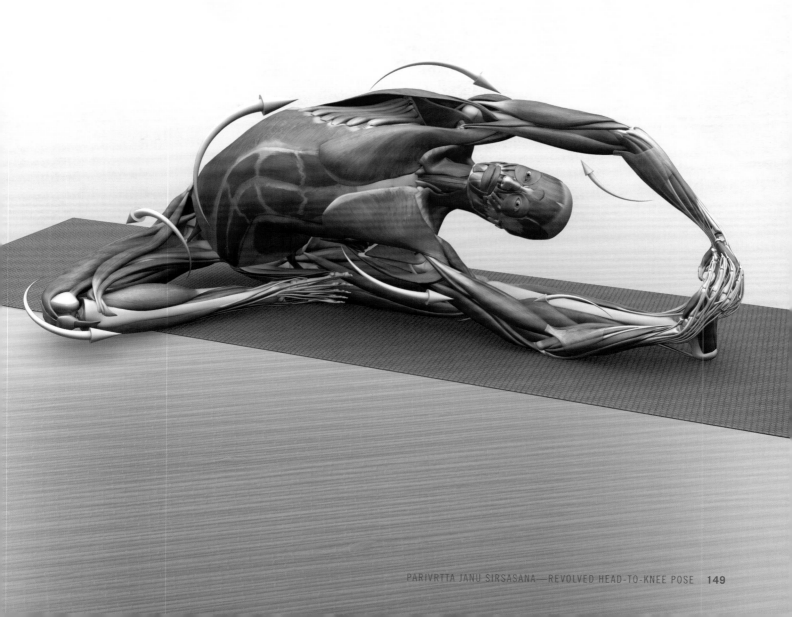

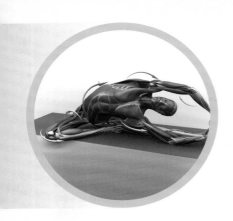

Parivrtta Janu Sirsasana Preparation

Use a belt to lasso the foot of the extended leg and laterally flex the torso over the thigh. Raise both arms over the head, and bend the elbows. Then begin to straighten the knee to draw the torso further over the leg. As you gain flexibility, reach forward and grasp the foot with the hands. You may need to start with the knee bent for this variation. Firmly grip the foot, and then contract the quadriceps to straighten the knee. Use the bent leg and hip to anchor the pelvis back while the torso flexes forward.

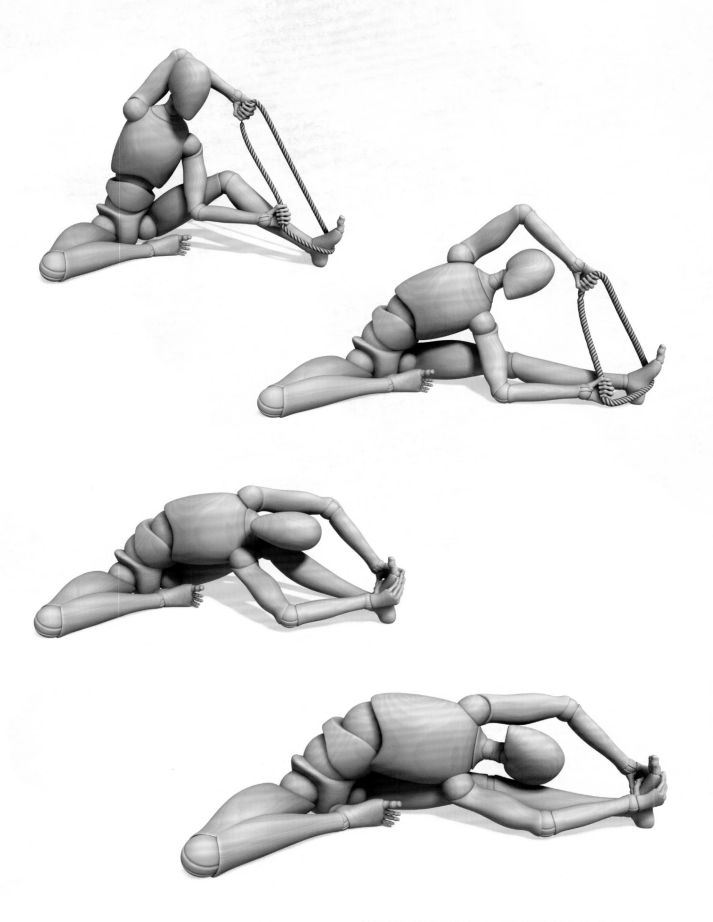

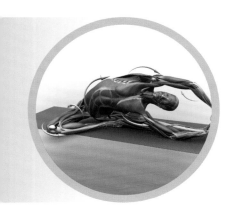

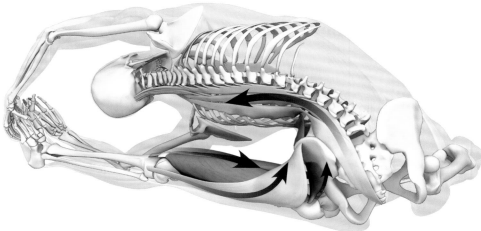

STEP 1 Engage the quadriceps to straighten the knee of the extended leg. Use the tensor fascia lata on the side of the leg to synergize this action. This muscle also flexes and internally rotates the thigh. The gluteus minimus, located deep to the tensor fascia lata, synergizes these actions. Visualize this muscle contracting. The quadriceps create reciprocal inhibition of the hamstrings, and the flexion component of the tensor fascia lata and gluteus minimus combines with the psoas to produce reciprocal inhibition of the gluteus maximus.

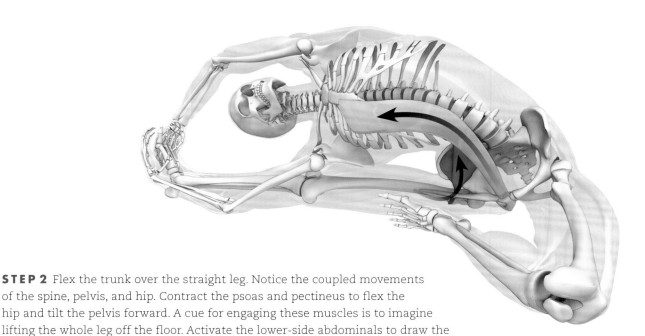

STEP 2 Flex the trunk over the straight leg. Notice the coupled movements of the spine, pelvis, and hip. Contract the psoas and pectineus to flex the hip and tilt the pelvis forward. A cue for engaging these muscles is to imagine lifting the whole leg off the floor. Activate the lower-side abdominals to draw the trunk against the thigh. Observe how this interacts with the ischial tuberosity at the back of the pelvis, creating one vertex of the triangle that focuses the stretch on the hamstrings. The insertion of the hamstrings is the other vertex of the triangle. Contract the quadriceps (see Step 1) to extend the knee, moving the insertions of the hamstrings away from their origin. Co-activate the muscles on the lower side of the trunk with the quadriceps to focus the stretch on the back of the extended leg.

▶ **STEP 3** The sartorius flexes, abducts, and externally rotates the hip of the bent leg. The hamstrings flex the knee. Engage both muscles to produce these actions, and be aware of how this affects the stretch on the upper side of the trunk. There is a tendency to neglect the bent leg while we focus on grasping the foot and stretching the straight leg. The position of the back leg, however, is an integral part of the pose—it produces a backward-directed force that deepens the stretch of the forward-flexing trunk.

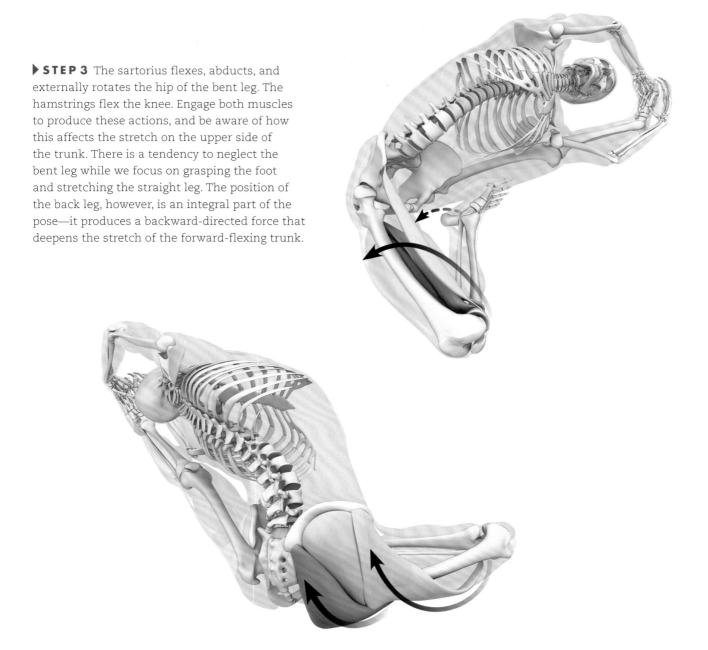

STEP 4 The abductors and external rotators of the hip (located deep to the gluteus maximus) synergize the actions of the sartorius and hamstrings. Contract the gluteus maximus to externally rotate the femur, and engage the deep external rotators to tuck the tailbone under. The tensor fascia lata and gluteus medius abduct the thigh. Although the main position of the femur is external rotation, the tensor fascia lata and gluteus medius also produce an internal rotation component that aids to protect the knee. Squeeze the lower leg against the upper leg by engaging the hamstrings, and turn the femur as one unit. Draw the thigh back and down diagonally, so that the knee joint is maintained as a hinge. Notice how these actions stabilize the pose by grounding the hip and pelvis.

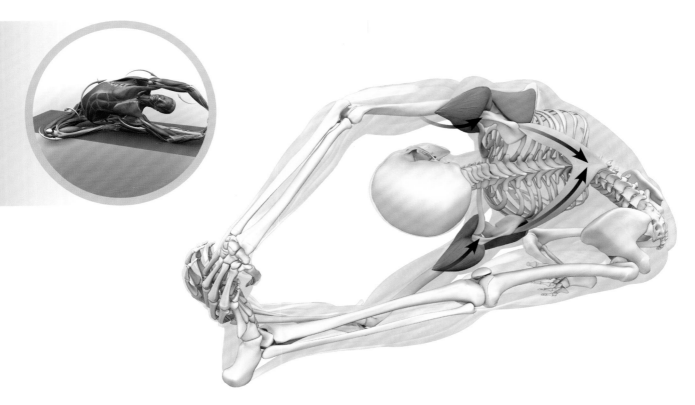

▲ **STEP 5** Press the back of the lower arm against the inside of the lower leg by contracting the deltoids. This action connects the upper and lower body. Because the arm is fixed against the thigh, engaging the deltoids rotates the trunk instead of moving the arm. Externally rotate the upper arm by activating the infraspinatus and teres minor muscles. Turning the shoulders in this way creates a "coiling" effect down the arms and into the hands (which are gripping the foot). Combine this with drawing the shoulders away from the neck by contracting the lower third of the trapezius. Note how this turns the chest forward. Arch the back by engaging the erector spinae and quadratus lumborum muscles (especially on the lower side).

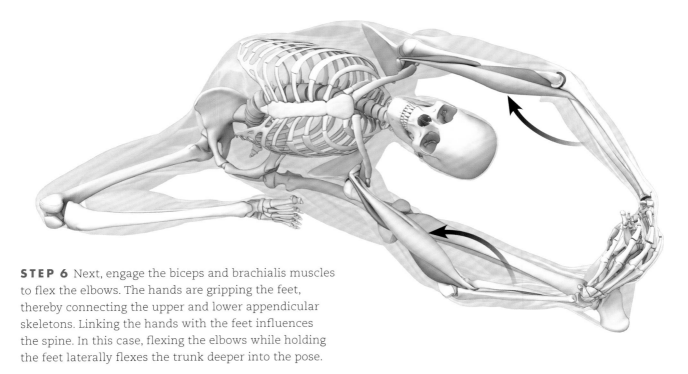

STEP 6 Next, engage the biceps and brachialis muscles to flex the elbows. The hands are gripping the feet, thereby connecting the upper and lower appendicular skeletons. Linking the hands with the feet influences the spine. In this case, flexing the elbows while holding the feet laterally flexes the trunk deeper into the pose.

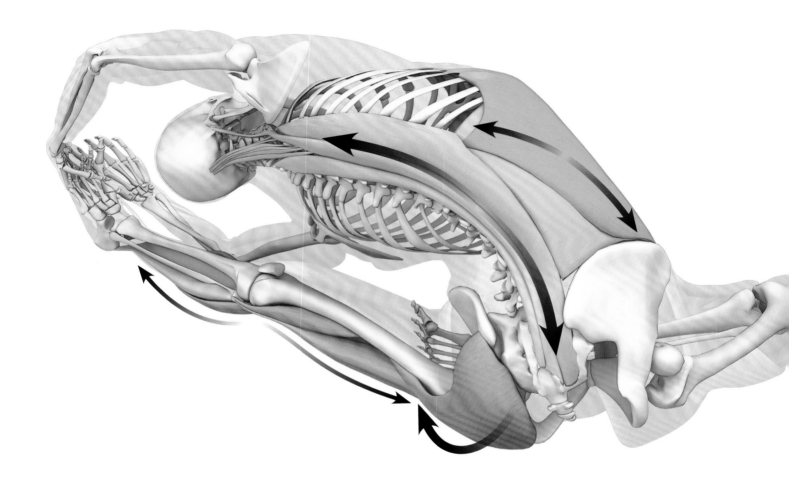

SUMMARY All of these actions orchestrate a deep stretch of the muscles at the back of the straight leg, including the gastrocnemius/soleus complex, the hamstrings, and the gluteus maximus. The upper-side erector spinae, quadratus lumborum, and various spinal rotators all lengthen as well. Additionally, the upper-side oblique and transverse abdominals stretch. Engage the lower-side erector spinae and abdominal muscles to flex the trunk deeper and accentuate the stretch.

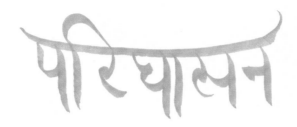

PARIGHASANA I
CROSS BAR OF THE GATE POSE VERSION I

PARIGHASANA I RESEMBLES PARIVRTTA JANU SIRSASANA IN THE POSITION OF the straight leg and trunk. It differs in that the bent-leg hip and thigh internally rotate (as opposed to externally rotating in Parivrtta Janu Sirsasana). The position of the bent leg has a ripple effect that spreads upward into the trunk and over to the straight leg. Abduct and extend the hip to create a direction of force backward through the bent knee. Note that this action tends to draw the torso towards that side and internally rotates the straight-leg thigh.

Use the external rotators of the straight leg to counteract this tendency and bring the kneecap back to neutral. Link the hand to the foot to connect the shoulders and pelvis through the spine. The laterally flexing chest and trunk produce an opposing energy that combines to stretch the side of the body and the back. The lower-side trunk engages and the upper side stretches. Balance and stabilize this action by eccentrically contracting the muscles of the upper side of the trunk, including the oblique abdominals and the quadratus lumborum. This stimulates a spinal cord reflex arc involving the Golgi tendon organ. After a few breaths, the muscles of the upper-side torso will relax. Take advantage of this to flex the trunk and turn the chest more deeply into the pose.

BASIC JOINT POSITIONS

- The bent-leg hip flexes, abducts, and internally rotates.
- The knee of the same leg flexes.
- The straight-leg hip flexes and externally rotates.
- The knee of the same leg extends.

- The trunk flexes and rotates.
- The shoulders abduct and flex.
- The elbows flex.
- The forearms supinate.
- The wrists flex.

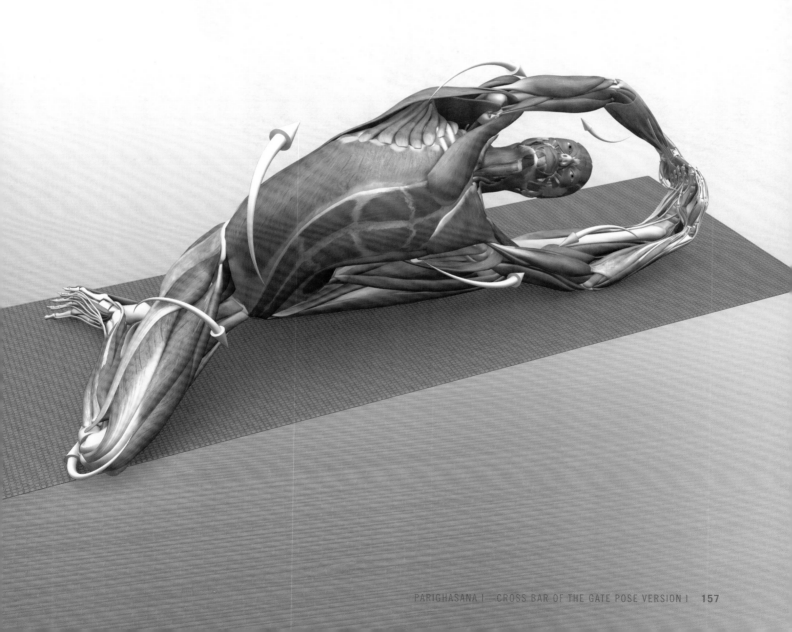

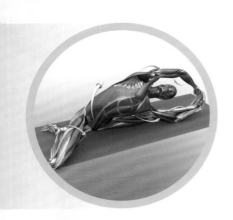

Parighasana I Preparation

Take the general shape of the pose and allow your body to acclimate before going deeper into the stretch. Remember that lengthening a muscle triggers a protective response from the spinal cord that actually causes that same muscle to contract. Holding a mild stretch (rather than a deep one) for a few breaths reassures the receptors in the muscle belly that you are stretching safely, so they decrease their firing, which allows the muscle to relax into the pose. Engaging the muscles that produce the general shape of Parighasana I, such as the straight-leg quadriceps and the lower-side oblique abdominals, also stimulates reciprocal inhibition of the muscles that are lengthening, accentuating their relaxation.

Loop a belt around the foot and flex the arms over the head. Bend the elbows and feel how this affects the trunk. Press out through the foot and feel this effect. Then combine these two actions. Engage the hamstring muscles to bend the other knee, and activate the tensor fascia lata and gluteus medius to internally rotate the hip. If you have knee pain, back off from the pose. Knee pain in this posture is usually caused by torque about the joint that takes it away from a hinge position and more into rotation. You may be able to counteract this by sitting on a block or blanket. As you gain flexibility, reach forward and firmly grasp the foot with the hands. Engage the quadriceps to straighten the knee and draw the trunk towards the thigh.

Your exit from this pose is as important as your entrance into it. Do not spring out of the asana. Plan your exit and ease out. For example, protect the hamstrings of the straight leg by slightly bending the knee before coming up. This releases the indirect pull on the hamstrings that results from the erector spinae contracting when you sit up out of the pose.

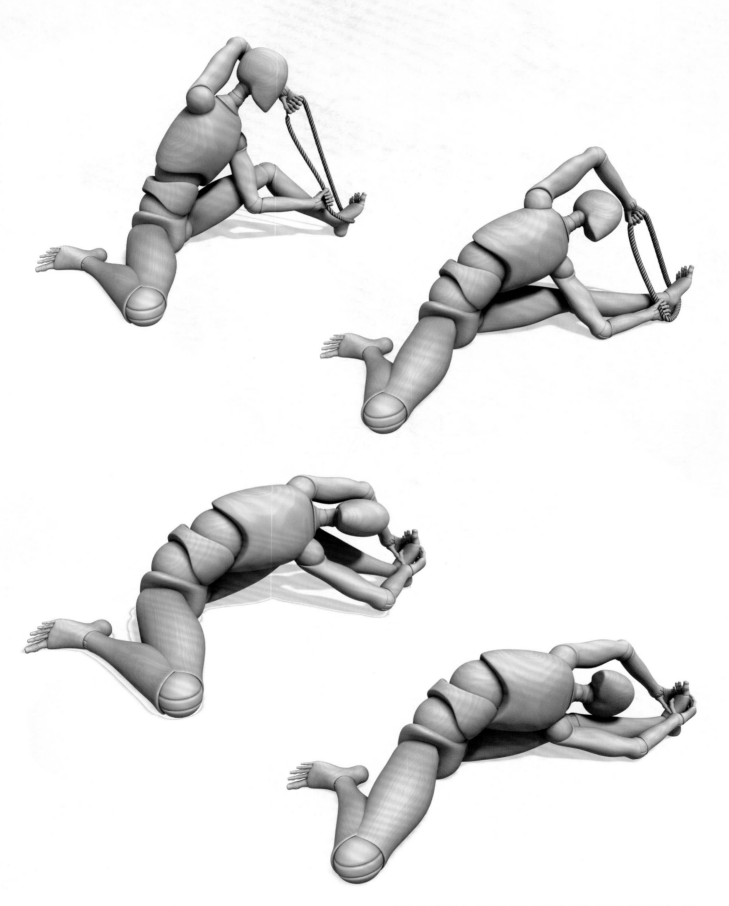

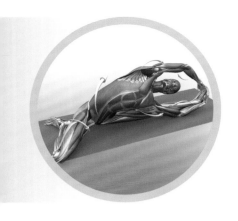

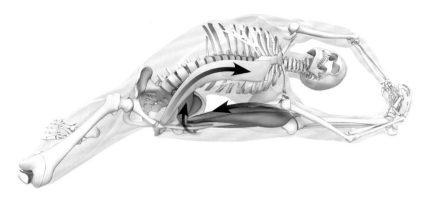

STEP 1 Engage the lower-side abdominals to flex the trunk over the straight leg. Combine this with activating the hip flexors, including the psoas and pectineus muscles. The cue for this action is to imagine lifting the entire leg off the floor while squeezing the trunk into the thigh. Straighten the knee by firmly engaging the quadriceps, and feel the anteversion of the pelvis. This is due to the contraction of the rectus femoris muscle pulling on the front of the ilium. Note how the stretch feels different when the quadriceps are fully engaged. This is because reciprocal inhibition causes the antagonist muscles, the hamstrings, to relax into the stretch.

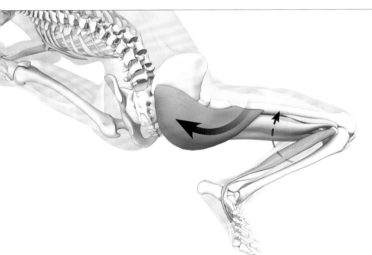

STEP 2 Extend the back hip by engaging the gluteus maximus. Contract the hamstrings to flex the knee, and activate the peroneus longus and brevis muscles to evert the foot (tilt it upward). Remember that engaging the gluteus maximus also externally rotates the hip. Step 3 balances this.

STEP 3 Engage the gluteus medius and tensor fascia lata to abduct the femur and internally rotate the thigh. This action helps to maintain congruency of the bent knee by moving it as a unit. There is a tendency for the inner side of the knee to open up in this position. Inwardly rotating the femur aids to counteract this.

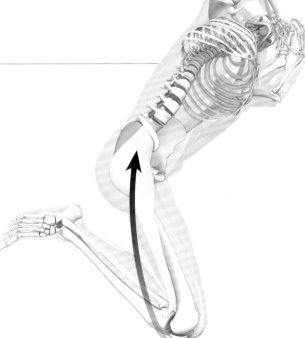

STEP 4 Contract the supinator muscle on the lower-side forearm to turn the palm up and the pronators teres and quadratus on the upper-side forearm to turn the mound of the index finger toward the foot. These actions lock the grip. Next, flex the elbows by contracting the biceps and brachialis muscles. Move up into the shoulders and engage the posterior deltoids to press the lower-side elbow against the knee and flex the upper-side elbow over the head. This rotates the body upward. Activate the infraspinatus and teres minor muscles of the rotator cuff to externally rotate both arms. The net effect of these actions is to draw the torso deeper into the pose and turn the chest towards the ceiling. Together the muscles of the arms and shoulders create a helical "coiling" effect, stabilizing the turn. Combine any of these actions with those in Step 1 to experience co-activation of muscles and create synergy between the upper and lower extremities.

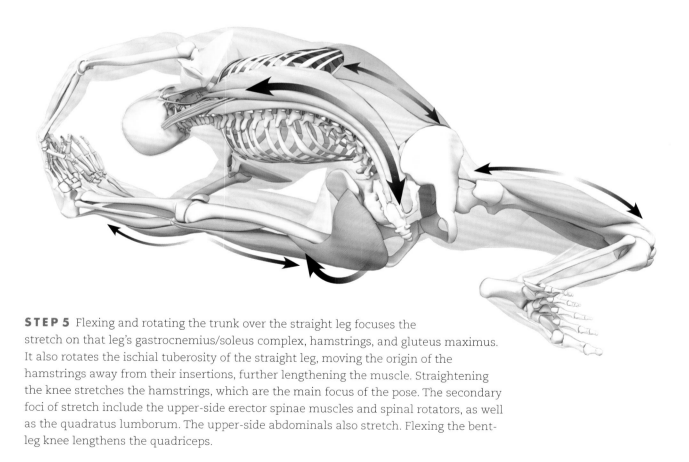

STEP 5 Flexing and rotating the trunk over the straight leg focuses the stretch on that leg's gastrocnemius/soleus complex, hamstrings, and gluteus maximus. It also rotates the ischial tuberosity of the straight leg, moving the origin of the hamstrings away from their insertions, further lengthening the muscle. Straightening the knee stretches the hamstrings, which are the main focus of the pose. The secondary foci of stretch include the upper-side erector spinae muscles and spinal rotators, as well as the quadratus lumborum. The upper-side abdominals also stretch. Flexing the bent-leg knee lengthens the quadriceps.

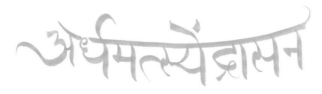

ARDHA MATSYENDRASANA

HALF LORD OF THE FISHES POSE

ARDHA MATSYENDRASANA CREATES THE SHAPE OF A FISH'S TAIL, WITH THE bottom knee flexing and the hip externally rotating. The upper leg has the foot crossed over the opposite thigh, with the knee and hip flexing. The main story of this pose involves turning the tail in the opposite direction of the upper body. Use points of contact between the upper and lower extremities to create this core movement. For example, whenever you have one part of the body fixed against another, as with the outside of the top-leg ankle against the thigh of the bottom leg, a point of leverage is created. Pressing the top-leg ankle against the thigh can be used as a cue for internally rotating the hip. The top knee is *adducting*, or moving across the midline, which means the *abductor* muscles (those that move the leg away from the midline) are stretching. A secondary action of the abductors is internal rotation of the femur. Pressing the ankle against the thigh eccentrically contracts the stretching abductors, internally rotating the hip—a desirable effect in this pose.

When you engage a muscle that is stretching, you stimulate the Golgi tendon organ. This causes the spinal cord to signal that same muscle to relax. In this example, the abductor muscles at the side of the hip relax and lengthen, allowing the knee to be drawn closer to the midline and turning the body deeper into the twist. Additionally, internally rotating the thigh stretches the deep external rotators of the hip. Ardha Matsyendrasana is one of the most effective poses for isolating these hard-to-access muscles. Internal rotation of the thigh is just one action in the pose. Look at the other points of contact—the back of the arm on the outer knee and the hand under the foot. You can use these points to deepen the posture.

Stability is gained from the core muscles of the pelvis. Note that the top hip is flexing relatively more than the bottom. Use the powerful hip flexors, including the psoas muscle, to accentuate this. Then contract the hip extensors and abductors to press the bottom-leg thigh into the floor. The hip flexors run along the inside of the pelvis and wrap over the front to insert onto the femur; the extensors run along the outside of the pelvis to insert on the outside of the femur. Engaging the hip flexors on one side of the pelvis and the extensors on the other side produces a "wringing" effect across the sacroiliac joint, creating tautness of the stout pelvic ligaments and ligamentotaxis. This stabilizes the foundation of the pose. As with other twists, connecting the upper and lower extremities deepens the turn of the vertebral column.

BASIC JOINT POSITIONS

- The hip of the leg that remains on the floor flexes, abducts, and externally rotates.
- The hip of the other leg flexes, adducts, and internally rotates.
- The knees flex.
- The trunk flexes and rotates.
- The shoulder of the arm behind the back extends and internally rotates.

- The elbow of the same arm flexes and the forearm supinates.
- The shoulder of the arm that holds the foot abducts and externally rotates.
- The elbow of the same arm flexes.
- The forearm pronates.
- The ankle of the foot that is held plantar flexes.

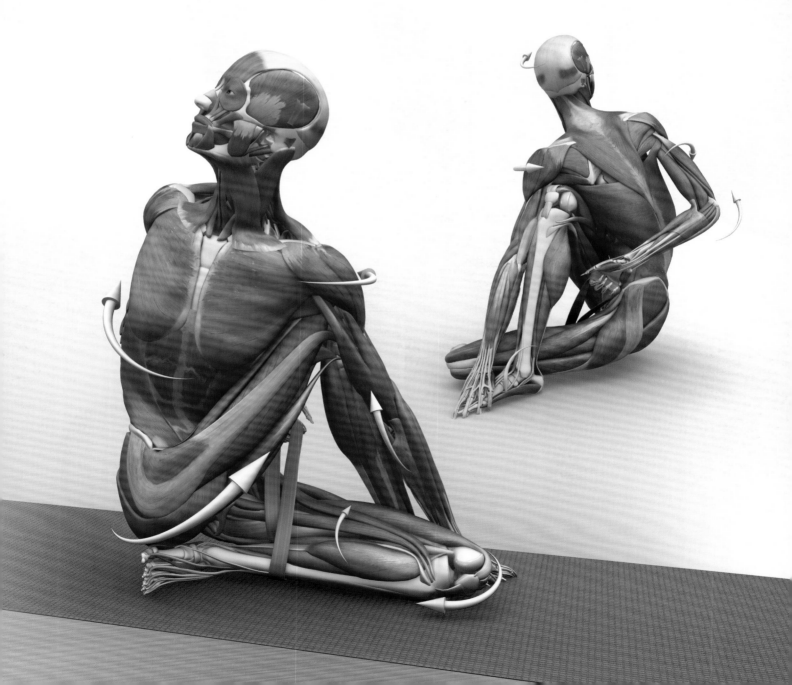

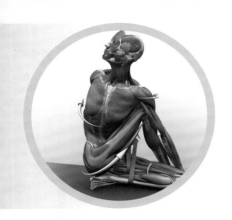

Ardha Matsyendrasana
Preparation

Begin by flexing the hip and knee and placing the foot on the outside of the opposite thigh. Wrap the opposite arm around the front of the knee, grasping it with the hand. Place the other hand on the floor behind the pelvis. Bend the elbow of the front arm and straighten the elbow of the arm that is on the floor. Activate the muscles of both arms simultaneously to turn the upper body.

As you gain flexibility, place the outside of the arm onto the outside of the flexed knee. Loop a belt around the lower leg, as shown, and grasp it with the hand that is behind the body. Press the elbow into the outer knee as you pull on the belt with the other hand. Feel how these actions combine to turn the torso.

The classical pose has the arm reaching forward around the side of the knee. Dorsiflex the foot (lift the sole of the foot off the ground while leaving the heel on the mat) and firmly grasp it with the hand. Then activate the calf muscles to plantar flex the foot. This presses the foot into the floor, drawing the hand with it and levering the body further into the twist.

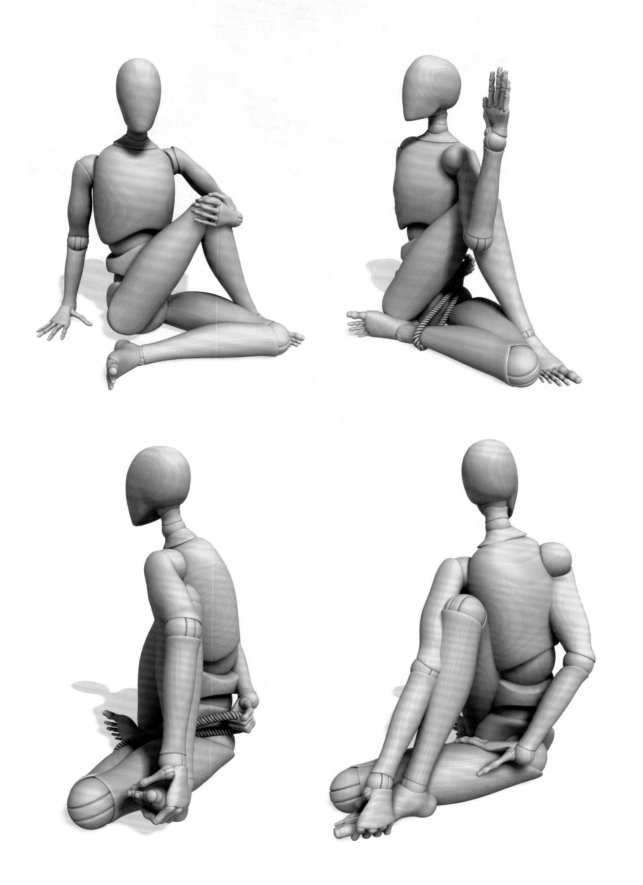

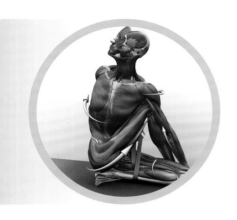

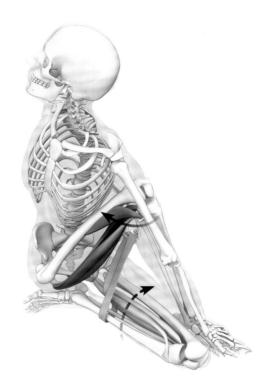

STEP 1 Bend both knees. The bottom knee is flexing more than the upper, so the hamstrings on this side will contract with greater force. Note that the tibia of the upper leg rotates externally. You can accentuate this by pressing the ball of the foot into the floor and gently turning it toward the outer edge of the mat. This engages the biceps femoris muscle on the outside of the thigh and rotates the tibia. Do this with caution. The force of the external rotation transmutes into internal rotation of the hip. This is accentuated by pressing the side of the knee into the elbow, engaging the gluteus medius and tensor fascia lata.

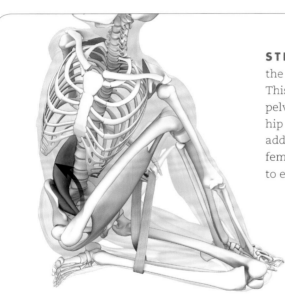

STEP 2 In Ardha Matsyendrasana, one knee flexes more than the other. Similarly, both hips flex, one more than the other. This produces an opportunity to create a bandha across the pelvis. Contract the upper-leg psoas and pectineus to flex the hip into the trunk and squeeze the trunk into the thigh. The adductors longus and brevis synergize this action and draw the femur across the midline. The psoas on the other leg engages to externally rotate the femur and tilts the pelvis forward.

STEP 3 Press the side of the thigh into the mat to engage the tensor fascia lata and gluteus medius muscles. Tuck the tailbone down and under to activate the gluteus maximus and deep external rotators, rolling the thigh outward.

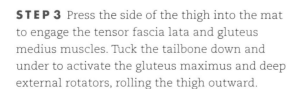

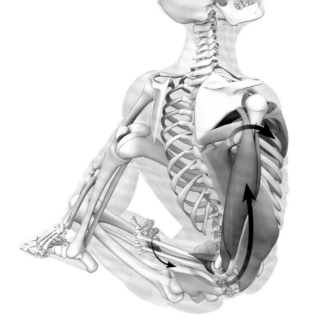

STEP 4 Roll the shoulder forward to internally rotate the arm behind the back. Lift the hand off the back to engage the muscles that produce this action. This causes the lower part of the pectoralis major, the latissimus dorsi, the teres major, the front part of the deltoid, and the subscapularis muscles to contract. Attempt to straighten the elbow by engaging the triceps. Note that as the elbow extends, the body turns deeper into the pose. Accentuate this action by engaging the pronators teres and quadratus to pronate the forearm.

STEP 5 Activate the pronators teres and quadratus to turn the palm down, locking the hand onto the foot. Then attempt to bend the elbow by contracting the biceps and brachialis muscles. This draws the shoulder and trunk deeper into the twist. It also aids to protect the elbow from hyperextension, which is the tendency in this pose.

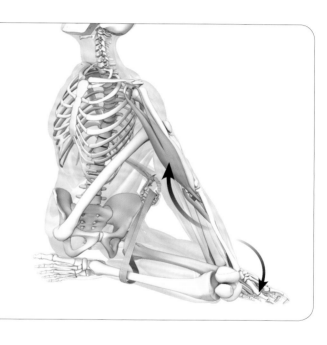

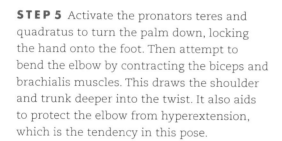

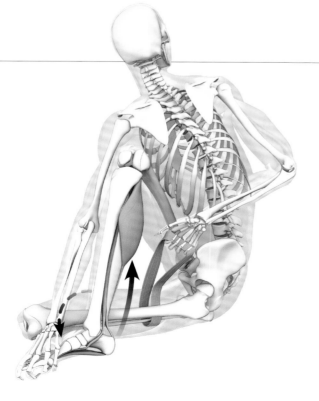

STEP 6 Plantar flex the foot (press it into the floor) by contracting the gastrocnemius/soleus complex, the flexor digitorum, the flexors hallucis longus and brevis, and the intrinsic flexors of the foot. This will draw the arm further forward and turn the body deeper into the twist.

RESTORATIVE POSES
SUPINE TWIST

Use a passive twist to release and restore the back muscles when cooling down from backbends. These images illustrate a twisting stretch of the lower back muscles and hip abductors. Cross the foot on the knee and then turn the pelvis as shown. Abduct the shoulders and turn the palms to face up. Turn the head.

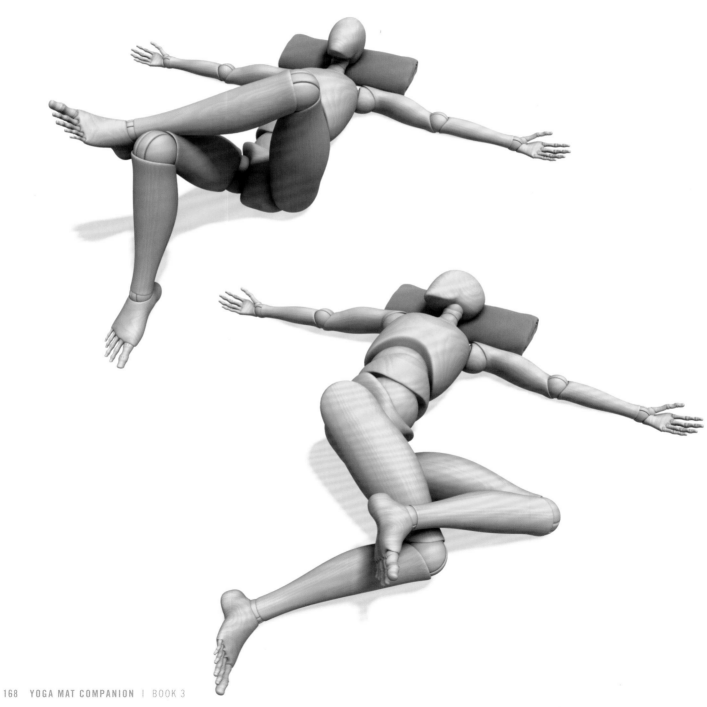

PROP TWIST

Practice a seated twist with a chair to release the upper back and shoulders. Place a blanket on the chair and then rest the head on the seat, as shown. Do the same with the chair to the side, turning this into a forward-bending twist. For a deeper variation, sit in Easy Cross-Legged Pose and bend forward to place the head on a block. Turn the trunk to make this a seated forward-bending twist. Then relax in Savasana.

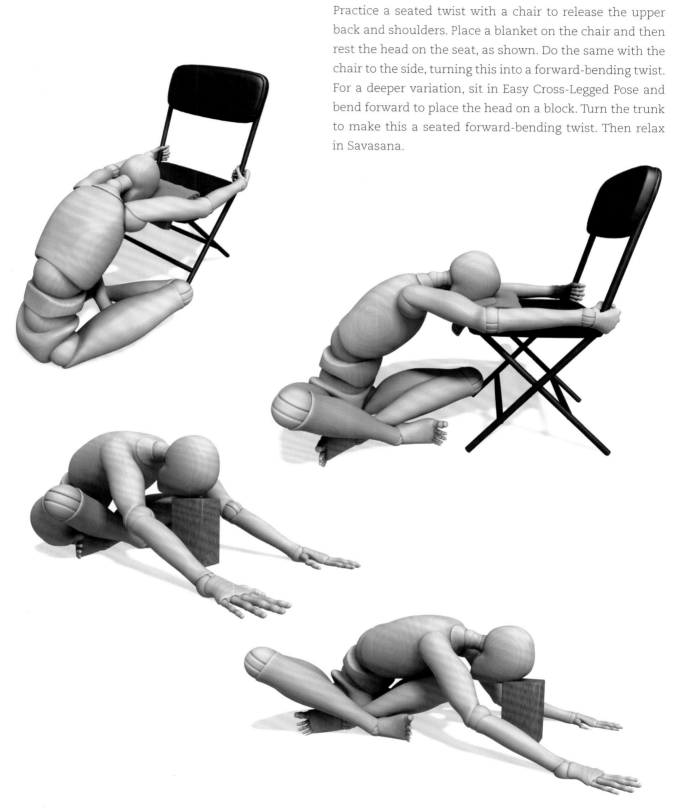

MOVEMENT
INDEX

MOVEMENT INDEX

Movements of the body have specific names. It is important to learn these names, both for teaching others yoga and for analyzing the muscles that produce the positions of the body. As a yoga teacher, it is always better to communicate your instructions in terminology that students can easily understand. Know the scientific names of the movements and have clear explanations to describe the movements in layperson's terms. Make your instructions as precise and uncomplicated as you can.

Remember that muscles contract to position the joints and appendages in the pose. If you know the joint positions, you can analyze which muscles to engage to produce the asana. With this knowledge comes the ability to use precise cues to communicate how to sculpt and stabilize the body in the pose, stretch the correct muscles, and create bandhas. Thus, unlocking the asana begins with a clear understanding of body movements.

There are six basic movements of the body: Flexion, Extension, Adduction, Abduction, Internal Rotation, and External Rotation. These movements take place in three planes, as shown here. The anatomic position is the reference point to define the direction of movement.

CORONAL PLANE: divides the body into front and back. Movements along this plane are called adduction and abduction. Adduction moves the extremity towards the midline and abduction moves the extremity away from the midline.

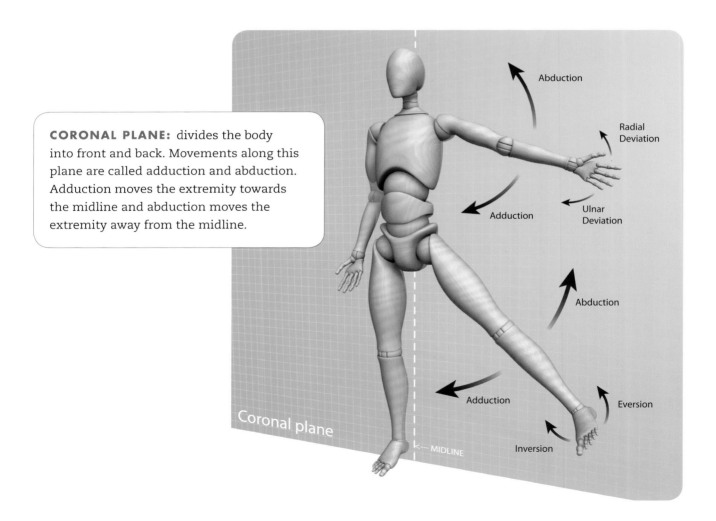

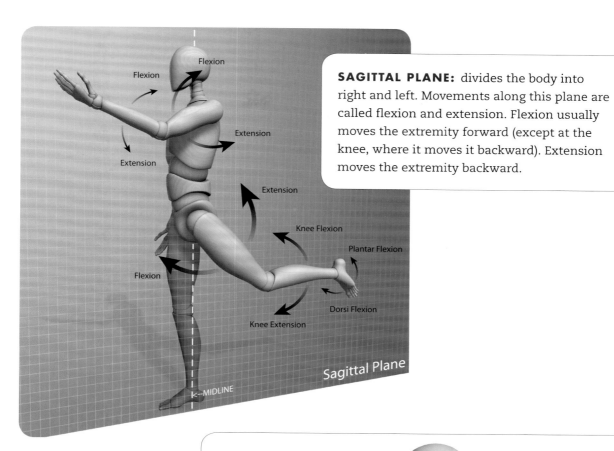

Flexion

Flexion

Extension

Extension

Extension

Flexion

Knee Flexion

Plantar Flexion

Dorsi Flexion

Knee Extension

Flexion

←MIDLINE

Sagittal Plane

SAGITTAL PLANE: divides the body into right and left. Movements along this plane are called flexion and extension. Flexion usually moves the extremity forward (except at the knee, where it moves it backward). Extension moves the extremity backward.

TRANSVERSE PLANE: divides the body into upper and lower halves. Movement along this plane is called rotation. Rotation is further classified as internal (towards the midline) and external (away from the midline). Internal and external rotation are also referred to as medial and lateral rotation, respectively.

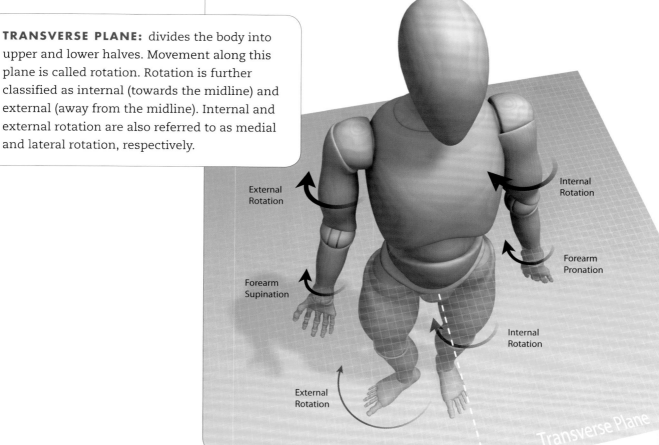

External Rotation

Internal Rotation

Forearm Pronation

Forearm Supination

Internal Rotation

External Rotation

Transverse Plane

MOVEMENT INDEX

Supta Padangusthasana, revolving version, and Natarajasana are presented as examples of how to analyze the basic joint positions in a yoga pose. The order represents the sequence of movements that create the form of the pose.

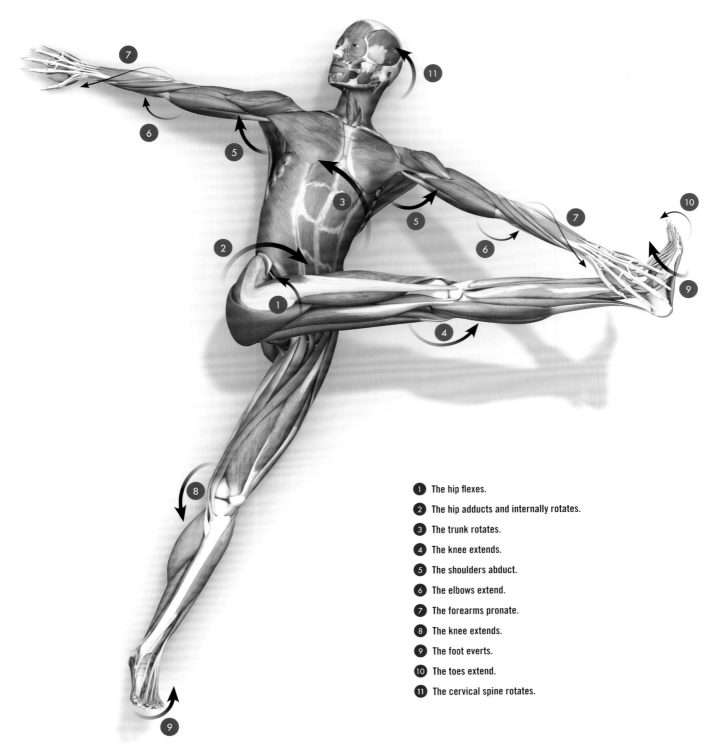

1. The hip flexes.
2. The hip adducts and internally rotates.
3. The trunk rotates.
4. The knee extends.
5. The shoulders abduct.
6. The elbows extend.
7. The forearms pronate.
8. The knee extends.
9. The foot everts.
10. The toes extend.
11. The cervical spine rotates.

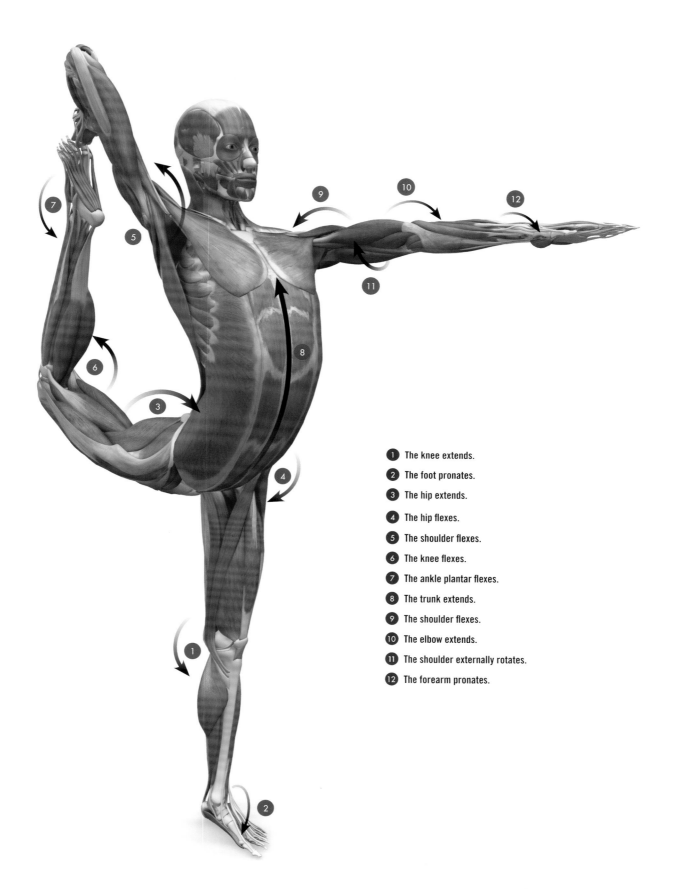

1 The knee extends.

2 The foot pronates.

3 The hip extends.

4 The hip flexes.

5 The shoulder flexes.

6 The knee flexes.

7 The ankle plantar flexes.

8 The trunk extends.

9 The shoulder flexes.

10 The elbow extends.

11 The shoulder externally rotates.

12 The forearm pronates.

MOVEMENT TABLES

Neck

Muscle	Flexion	Extension	Lateral Flexion	Lateral Extension	Rotation
Semispinalis capitis		●	●	●	●
Splenius capitis		●	●	●	●
Sternocleidomastoid	●		●	●	●
Levator scapulae		●	●	●	
Trapezius		●	●	●	●

Trunk

Muscle	Flexion	Extension	Lateral Flexion	Rotation
External oblique	●		●	●
Internal oblique	●		●	●
Rectus abdominis	●			
Spinalis thoracis		●		
Lateral intertransversi			●	
Interspinales		●		
Longissimus thoracis		●		
Iliocostalis lumborum		●		
Multifidus		●		
Rotatores		●		●
Quadratus lumborum		●	●	
Psoas major	●		●	
Iliacus	●		●	

Hip

Muscle	Flexion	Extension	Adduction	Abduction	Internal Rotation	External Rotation
Gluteus maximus		●				●
Gluteus medius	●	●		●	●	●
Gluteus minimus	●	●		●	●	●
Tensor fascia lata	●			●	●	
Psoas major	●					●
Iliacus	●					●
Rectus femoris	●			●		
Sartorius	●			●		●
Pectineus	●		●			●
Adductor magnus		●	●			●
Adductor longus	●		●			●
Adductor brevis	●		●			●
Gracilis	●		●			●
Piriformis				●		●
Gemellus superior				●		●
Gemellus inferior				●		●
Obturator internus				●		●
Obturator externus						●
Quadratus femoris			●			●
Semitendinosus		●			●	
Semimembranosus		●			●	
Biceps femoris		●				●

MOVEMENT TABLES

Knee

Muscle	Flexion	Extension	Internal Rotation	External Rotation
Vastus medialis		●		
Vastus lateralis		●		
Vastus intermedius		●		
Rectus femoris		●		
Sartorius	●			●
Semitendinosus	●		●	
Semimembranosus	●		●	
Biceps femoris	●			●
Gracilis	●		●	
Popliteus	●			
Gastrocnemius	●			

Lower Leg

Muscle	Ankle Plantar Flexion	Ankle Dorsiflexion	Foot Eversion	Foot Inversion	Toe Flexion	Toe Extension
Gastrocnemius	●					
Soleus	●					
Tibialis anterior		●		●		
Tibialis posterior	●			●		
Peroneus longus	●		●			
Peroneus brevis	●		●			
Peroneus tertius	●		●			
Flexor digitorum longus	●			●	●	
Flexor hallucis longus	●			●	●	
Extensor digitorum longus		●	●			●
Extensor hallucis longus		●		●		●

Foot

Muscle	Toe Flexion	Toe Extension	Toe Adduction	Toe Abduction
Flexor digitorum brevis	●			
Flexor hallucis brevis	●			
Flexor digiti minimi brevis	●			
Extensor digitorum brevis		●		
Extensor hallucis brevis		●		
Abductor digiti minimi				●
Abductor hallucis				●
Adductor hallucis			●	
Lumbricales	●	●	●	
Plantar interosseus	●		●	
Dorsal interosseus	●			●

Hand

Muscle	Flexion	Extension	Adduction	Abduction
Flexor digitorum superficialis	●			
Flexor digitorum profundus	●			
Flexor pollicis longus	●			
Flexor pollicis brevis	●			
Flexor digiti minimi brevis	●			
Extensor digitorum		●		
Extensor pollicis longus		●		
Extensor pollicis brevis		●		
Extensor indicis		●		
Extensor digiti minimi		●		
Abductor pollicis longus				●
Abductor pollicis brevis				●
Adductor pollicis			●	
Abductor digiti minimi				●
Lumbricales	●	●		
Dorsal interosseus	●	●	●	

MOVEMENT TABLES

Arm and Wrist

Muscle	Elbow Flexion	Elbow Extension	Forearm Pronation	Forearm Supination	Wrist Flexion	Wrist Extension	Wrist Ulnar Deviation	Wrist Radial Deviation
Biceps brachii	●			●				
Brachialis	●							
Triceps brachii		●						
Anconeus		●						
Brachioradialis	●							
Supinator				●				
Pronator teres			●					
Pronator quadratus			●					
Extensor carpi radialis longus						●		●
Extensor carpi radialis brevis						●		●
Extensor carpi ulnaris						●	●	
Flexor carpi radialis					●			●
Flexor carpi ulnaris					●		●	
Extensor digitorum						●		
Extensor pollicis brevis								●
Extensor pollicis longus				●				●
Abductor pollicis longus								●

Shoulder

Muscle	Retraction	Protraction	Elevation	Depression	Flexion	Extension	Adduction	Abduction	Internal Rotation	External Rotation
Rhomboids	●									
Serratus anterior		●	●					●		
Trapezius	●		●	●			●	●		
Levator scapulae		●	●							
Latissimus dorsi	●			●		●	●		●	
Teres major						●	●		●	
Pectoralis major				●	●		●		●	
Pectoralis minor		●		●						
Anterior deltoid					●				●	
Lateral deltoid								●		
Posterior deltoid						●				●
Supraspinatus								●		
Infraspinatus										●
Teres minor							●			●
Subscapularis									●	
Biceps brachii					●					
Coracobrachialis					●		●			
Triceps brachii						●	●			

ANATOMY
INDEX

ANATOMY INDEX
BONES

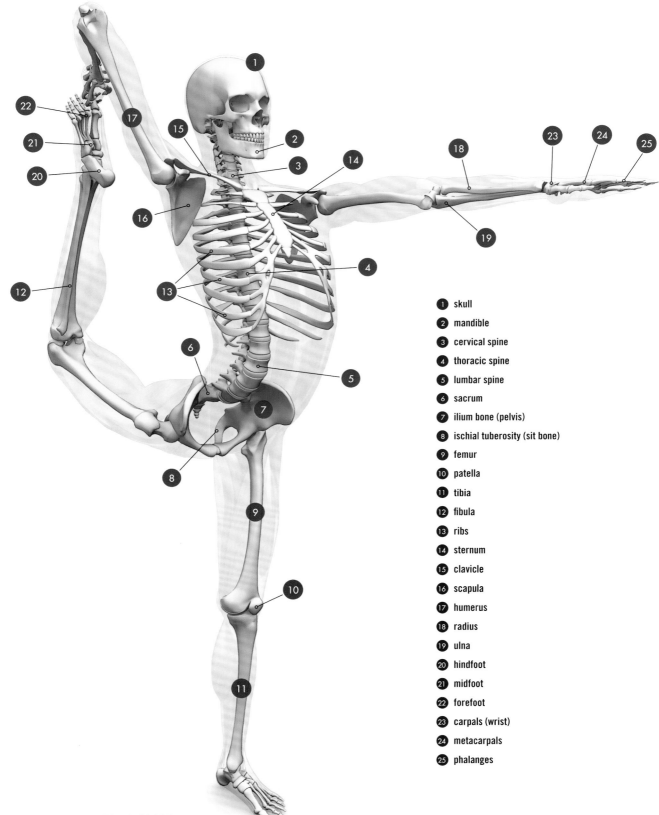

1. skull
2. mandible
3. cervical spine
4. thoracic spine
5. lumbar spine
6. sacrum
7. ilium bone (pelvis)
8. ischial tuberosity (sit bone)
9. femur
10. patella
11. tibia
12. fibula
13. ribs
14. sternum
15. clavicle
16. scapula
17. humerus
18. radius
19. ulna
20. hindfoot
21. midfoot
22. forefoot
23. carpals (wrist)
24. metacarpals
25. phalanges

AXIAL AND APPENDICULAR SKELETONS

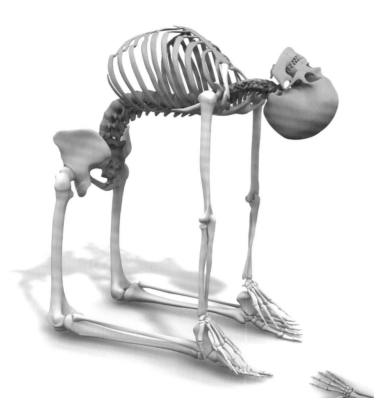

AXIAL SKELETON
The axial skeleton is composed of the skull, spine, and ribcage. It links the upper and lower appendicular skeletons. Thus, the two subdivisions can be used to affect and influence each other.

For example, in Ustrasana, connecting the hands to the soles of the feet aids in extending the spine.

APPENDICULAR SKELETON
The upper appendicular skeleton is composed of the shoulder (pectoral) girdle and the upper extremities. The shoulder girdle, which is composed of the scapula and clavicle, connects the arm to the trunk and thereby links the upper appendicular skeleton to the axial skeleton.

The lower appendicular skeleton is composed of the pelvic girdle and lower extremities. The pelvic girdle is composed of the iliac bones, the ischia, the pubic bones, and the pubic symphysis. The pelvic girdle connects the lower extremities to the axial skeletons.

It is important to understand the subdivisions of the skeleton because the appendicular skeleton can be used to leverage and move the axial skeleton. Put another way, connecting the hand to the foot affects the spine.

For example, pressing the hand onto the outside of the ankle in Supta Padangusthasana, revolving version, aids to turn the trunk.

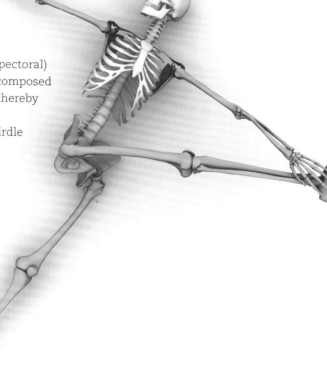

ANATOMY INDEX
MUSCLES

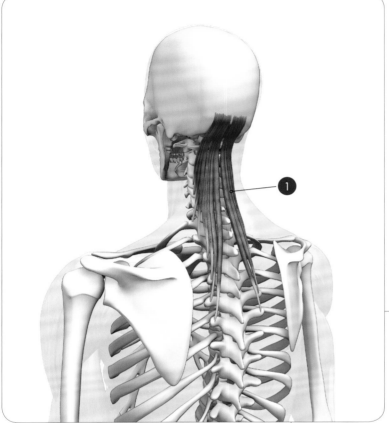

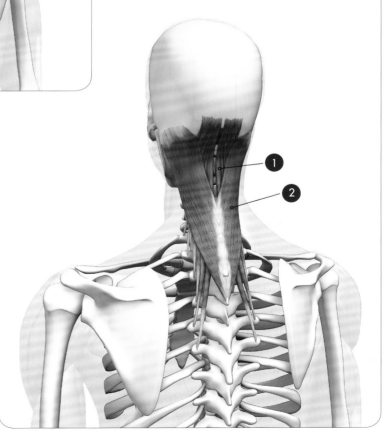

1 Semispinalis capitis

O: Transverse processes of lower cervical and upper thoracic vertebrae.

I: Occipital bone.

A: Extends head (tilts it back), assists in turning head.

2 Splenius capitis

O: Spinous processes of C7 and T1-4.

I: Mastoid process of skull, behind ear.

A: Extends head and neck; when one side contracts, laterally flexes neck; turns head toward side of individual muscle.

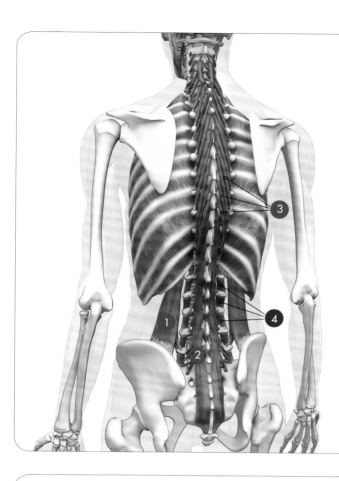

1 **Quadratus lumborum**

O: Posterior (back) of iliac crest.

I: Back part of rib 12, transverse processes of L1-4.

A: Laterally flexes spine (bends to side); extends and stabilizes lumbar spine; stabilizes rib 12, drawing it down during deep inhalation.

2 **Multifidus**

O: Back of sacrum and posterior superior iliac spine, transverse processes of lumbar, thoracic, and cervical vertebrae (all the way up the spine).

I: Two vertebrae above the vertebrae of origin; fibers are directed diagonally toward the midline and onto the spinous processes of the vertebrae of insertion.

A: Stabilizes spine during extension, flexion, and rotation.

3 **Semispinalis thoracis**

O: Transverse processes of T6-10.

I: Spinous processes of lower cervical and upper thoracic vertebrae.

A: Extends and rotates upper thoracic and lower cervical spine.

4 **Lateral intertransversi**

O: Transverse processes of lumbar vertebrae.

I: Transverse process of vertebrae immediately above vertebrae of origin.

A: Laterally flexes lumbar spine.

---

1 **Serratus posterior superior**

O: Ligamentum nuchae and spinous processes of C7-T4.

I: Ribs 2-5 on upper border.

A: Expands back of chest during deep inhalation by lifting ribs (is an accessory muscle of breathing).

2 **Serratus posterior inferior**

O: Spinous processes of T11-12, L1-3, thoracolumbar fascia.

I: Lower borders of ribs 9-12.

A: Stabilizes lower ribs during inhalation.

3 **Spinalis thoracis**

O: Transverse processes of T6-10.

I: Spinous processes of C6-7, T1-4.

A: Extends upper thoracic and lower cervical spine.

4 **Longissimus thoracis**

O: Posterior sacrum, spinous processes of T11-12, L1-5.

I: Transverse processes of T1-12, medial part of ribs 4-12.

A: Laterally flexes and extends spine, aids to expand chest during inhalation.

5 **Iliocostalis lumborum**

O: Posterior sacrum.

I: Posterior part of ribs 7-12.

A: Laterally flexes and extends lumbar spine.

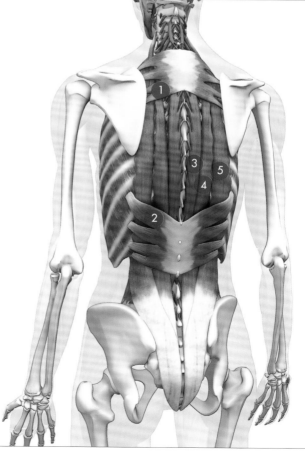

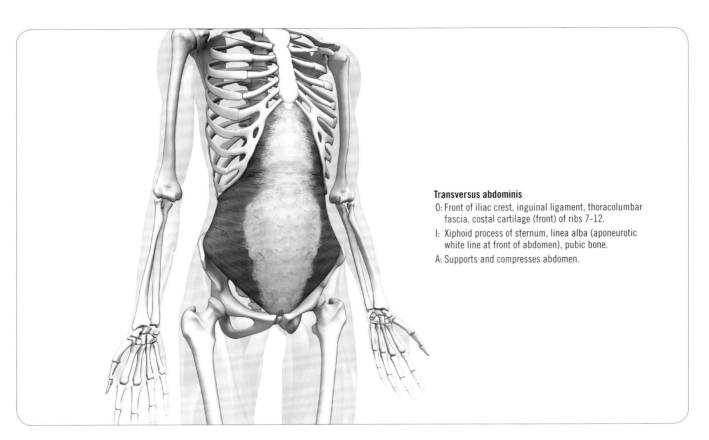

Transversus abdominis

O: Front of iliac crest, inguinal ligament, thoracolumbar fascia, costal cartilage (front) of ribs 7-12.

I: Xiphoid process of sternum, linea alba (aponeurotic white line at front of abdomen), pubic bone.

A: Supports and compresses abdomen.

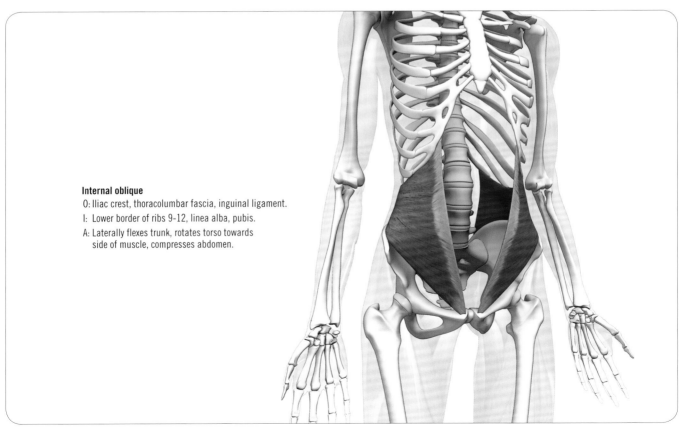

Internal oblique

O: Iliac crest, thoracolumbar fascia, inguinal ligament.

I: Lower border of ribs 9-12, linea alba, pubis.

A: Laterally flexes trunk, rotates torso towards side of muscle, compresses abdomen.

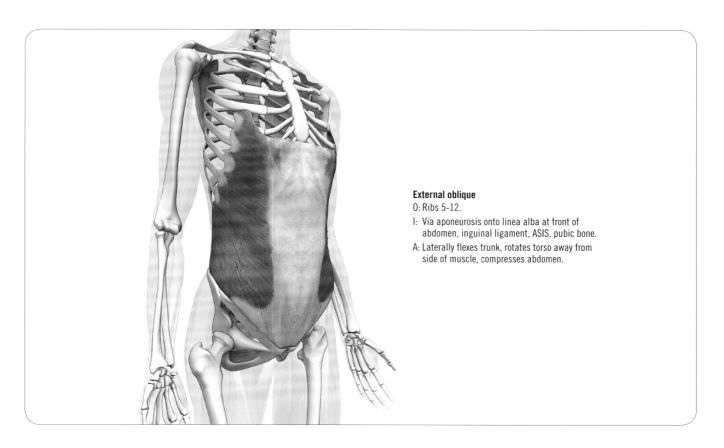

External oblique

O: Ribs 5-12.

I: Via aponeurosis onto linea alba at front of abdomen, inguinal ligament, ASIS, pubic bone.

A: Laterally flexes trunk, rotates torso away from side of muscle, compresses abdomen.

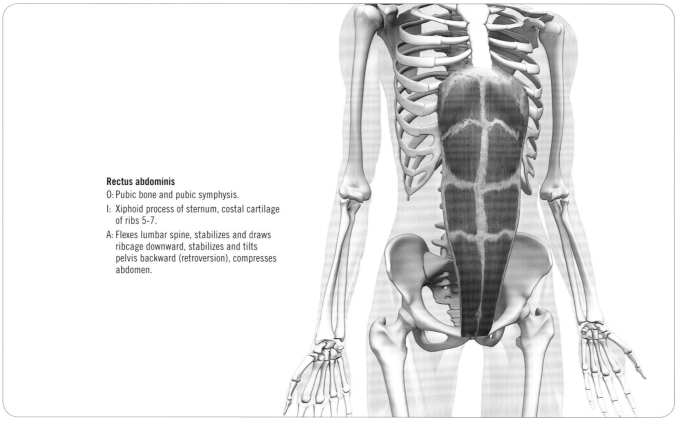

Rectus abdominis

O: Pubic bone and pubic symphysis.

I: Xiphoid process of sternum, costal cartilage of ribs 5-7.

A: Flexes lumbar spine, stabilizes and draws ribcage downward, stabilizes and tilts pelvis backward (retroversion), compresses abdomen.

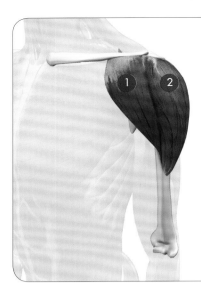

❶ Anterior deltoid
O: Front and top of lateral third of clavicle.
I: Deltoid tuberosity on outer surface of humeral shaft.
A: Forward flexes and internally rotates humerus.

❷ Lateral deltoid
O: Lateral border of acromion process of scapula.
I: Deltoid tuberosity on outer surface of humeral shaft.
A: Abducts humerus following initiation of movement by supraspinatus muscle of rotator cuff.

❸ Posterior deltoid
O: Spine of scapula.
I: Deltoid tuberosity on outer surface of humeral shaft.
A: Extends and externally rotates humerus.

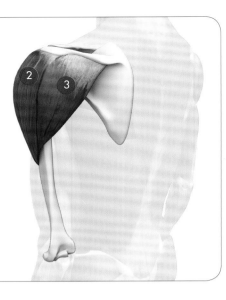

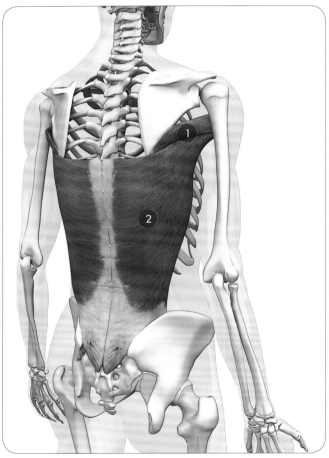

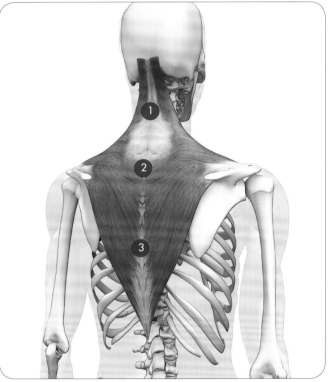

❶ Teres major
O: Lower lateral border of scapula.
I: Bicipital groove of humerus.
A: Adducts and internally rotates humerus.

❷ Latissimus dorsi
O: Thoracolumbar fascia, posterior portion of iliac crest, ribs 9-12, inferior border of scapula.
I: Bicipital groove of humerus.
A: Extends, adducts, and internally rotates humerus.

❶ Upper trapezius
O: Occipital bone, ligamentum nuchae.
I: Upper border of spine of scapula.
A: Elevates (lifts) shoulder girdle, with lower trapezius rotates scapula to lift arm overhead.

❷ Middle trapezius
O: Spinous processes of C7-T7.
I: Medial edge of acromion, posterior part of lateral third of clavicle.
A: Adducts (retracts) scapula.

❸ Lower trapezius
O: Spinous processes of T8-12.
I: Medial edge of acromion, posterior part of lateral third of clavicle.
A: Depresses scapula, aids to hold body in arm balancing, with upper trapezius rotates scapula to lift arm overhead.

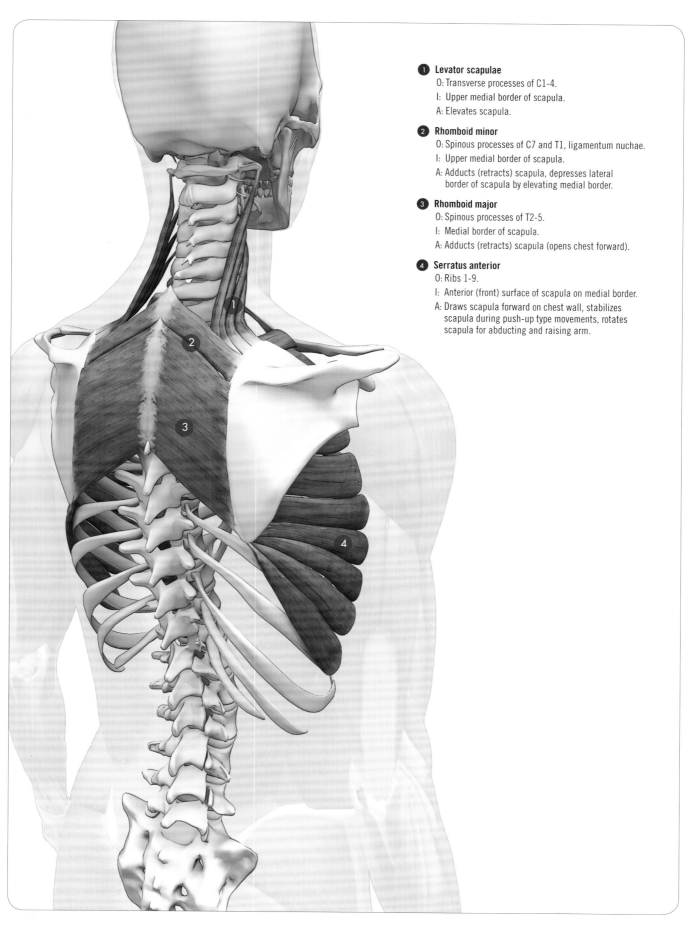

1 Levator scapulae
O: Transverse processes of C1-4.
I: Upper medial border of scapula.
A: Elevates scapula.

2 Rhomboid minor
O: Spinous processes of C7 and T1, ligamentum nuchae.
I: Upper medial border of scapula.
A: Adducts (retracts) scapula, depresses lateral border of scapula by elevating medial border.

3 Rhomboid major
O: Spinous processes of T2-5.
I: Medial border of scapula.
A: Adducts (retracts) scapula (opens chest forward).

4 Serratus anterior
O: Ribs 1-9.
I: Anterior (front) surface of scapula on medial border.
A: Draws scapula forward on chest wall, stabilizes scapula during push-up type movements, rotates scapula for abducting and raising arm.

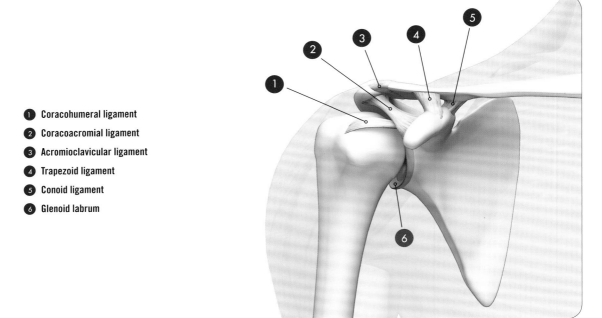

1. Coracohumeral ligament
2. Coracoacromial ligament
3. Acromioclavicular ligament
4. Trapezoid ligament
5. Conoid ligament
6. Glenoid labrum

1 Supraspinatus
O: Supraspinatus fossa of scapula.
I: Greater tuberosity of humerus.
A: Initiates abduction of humerus (raising arm to side),
stabilizes head of humerus in socket of shoulder joint.

2 Subscapularis
O: Front surface of scapula in subscapular fossa.
I: Lesser tuberosity of humerus.
A: Internally rotates humerus, stabilizes head
of humerus in socket of shoulder joint.

3 Teres minor
O: Upper part of lateral border of scapula.
I: Back and lower part of greater tuberosity of humerus.
A: Externally rotates humerus, stabilizes head
of humerus in socket of shoulder joint.

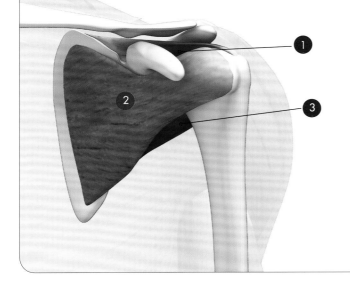

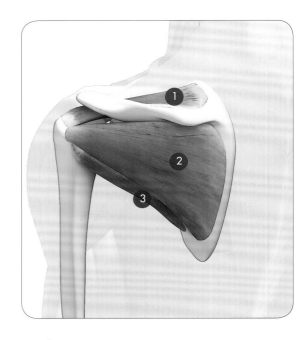

1 Supraspinatus
O: Supraspinatus fossa of scapula.
I: Greater tuberosity of humerus.
A: Initiates abduction of humerus (raising arm to side),
stabilizes head of humerus in socket of shoulder joint.

2 Infraspinatus
O: Infraspinatus fossa of scapula.
I: Greater tuberosity of humerus.
A: Externally rotates shoulder.

3 Teres minor
O: Upper part of lateral border of scapula.
I: Back and lower part of greater tuberosity of humerus.
A: Externally rotates humerus, stabilizes head
of humerus in socket of shoulder joint.

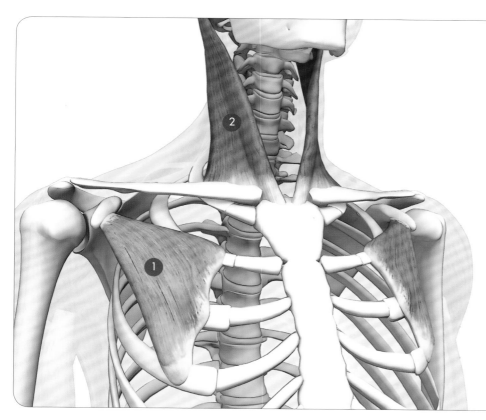

1 Pectoralis minor

O: Front of ribs 3-5.

I: Coracoid process of scapula.

A: Rolls shoulder forward and down (via scapula), lifts ribcage when scapula is stabilized by rhomboids (expands chest) through closed chain contraction.

2 Sternocleidomastoid

O: Sternal head: manubrium of sternum; clavicular head: upper surface of medial third of clavicle.

I: Mastoid process behind and below ear.

A: When both sides contract together flexes neck and tilts head forward; if head is stabilized, lifts upper ribcage during inhalation; contracting one side tilts head to side of muscle, rotates head to face away from muscle.

1 Pectoralis major

O: Sternocostal head: front of manubrium and body of sternum; clavicular head: medial half of clavicle.

I: Outer edge of bicipital groove on upper humerus.

A: Adducts and internally rotates humerus. Sternocostal head draws humerus down and across the body towards opposite hip. Clavicular head forward flexes and internally rotates the humerus, draws humerus across body towards opposite shoulder.

2 Coracobrachialis

O: Coracoid process of scapula.

I: Inner surface of humerus at mid-shaft.

A: Assists pectoralis in adduction of humerus and shoulder.

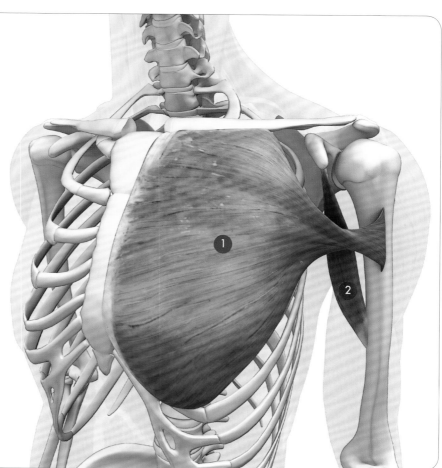

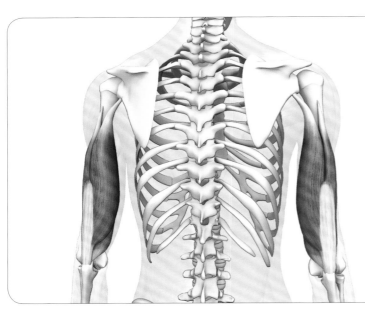

Triceps brachii

O: Long head from infraglenoid tubercle at bottom of shoulder socket; medial and lateral heads from posterior surface of humerus and intermuscular septum.

I: Olecranon process of ulna.

A: Extends elbow, long head moves arm back and adducts it.

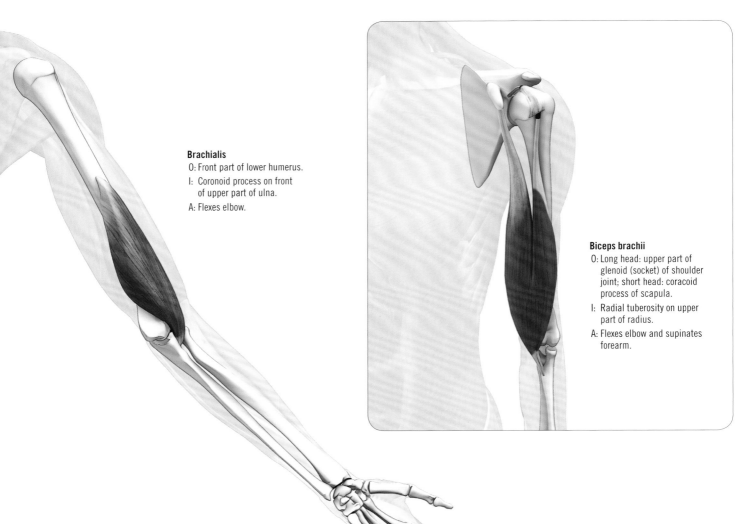

Brachialis

O: Front part of lower humerus.

I: Coronoid process on front of upper part of ulna.

A: Flexes elbow.

Biceps brachii

O: Long head: upper part of glenoid (socket) of shoulder joint; short head: coracoid process of scapula.

I: Radial tuberosity on upper part of radius.

A: Flexes elbow and supinates forearm.

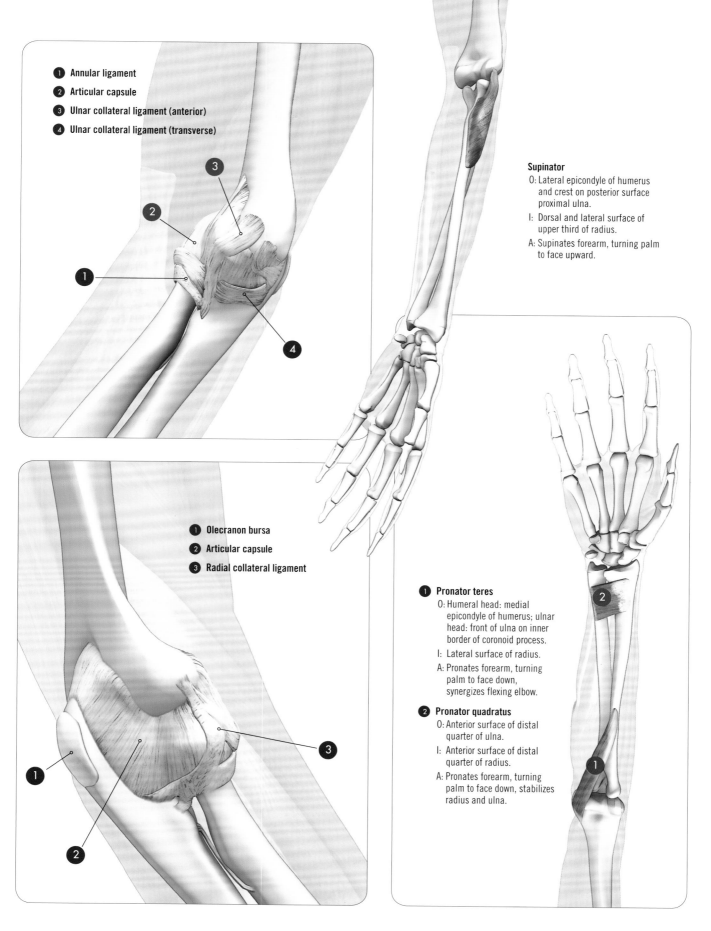

Annular ligament — 1
Articular capsule — 2
Ulnar collateral ligament (anterior) — 3
Ulnar collateral ligament (transverse) — 4

Supinator

O: Lateral epicondyle of humerus and crest on posterior surface proximal ulna.

I: Dorsal and lateral surface of upper third of radius.

A: Supinates forearm, turning palm to face upward.

Olecranon bursa — 1
Articular capsule — 2
Radial collateral ligament — 3

1 Pronator teres

O: Humeral head: medial epicondyle of humerus; ulnar head: front of ulna on inner border of coronoid process.

I: Lateral surface of radius.

A: Pronates forearm, turning palm to face down, synergizes flexing elbow.

2 Pronator quadratus

O: Anterior surface of distal quarter of ulna.

I: Anterior surface of distal quarter of radius.

A: Pronates forearm, turning palm to face down, stabilizes radius and ulna.

1 **Flexor digitorum profundis**

O: Upper two thirds of anterior and medial surface of ulna and interosseous membrane (between radius and ulna).

I: Palmar (anterior) surface of distal phalanges of fingers.

A: Flexes distal phalanges, synergizes flexion of more proximal phalanges and wrist.

2 **Flexor pollicis longus**

O: Anterior surface of mid-shaft of radius, coronoid process of ulna, medial epicondyle.

I: Palmar (anterior) surface of distal phalanx of thumb.

A: Flexes thumb and synergizes flexion of wrist.

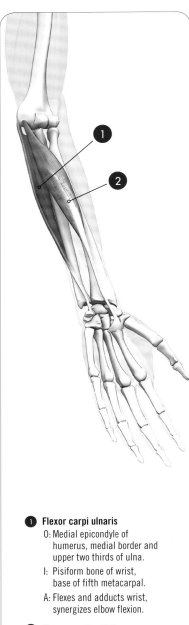

Flexor digitorum superficialis

O: Medial epicondyle, coronoid process of ulna, upper anterior border of radius.

I: Two slips of tendon insert onto either side of middle phalanges of four fingers.

A: Flexes middle phalanges of fingers, synergizes wrist flexion.

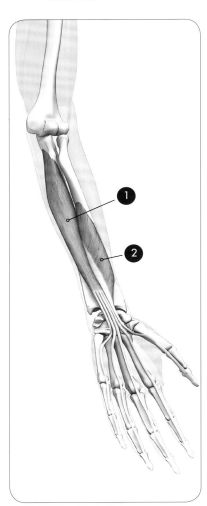

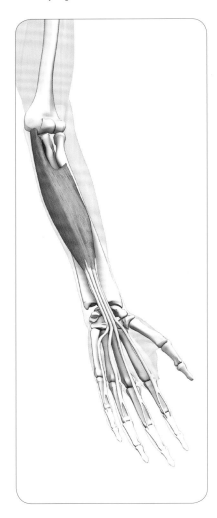

1 **Flexor carpi ulnaris**

O: Medial epicondyle of humerus, medial border and upper two thirds of ulna.

I: Pisiform bone of wrist, base of fifth metacarpal.

A: Flexes and adducts wrist, synergizes elbow flexion.

2 **Flexor carpi radialis**

O: Medial epicondyle of humerus.

I: Base of second metacarpal.

A: Flexes and abducts wrist, synergizes elbow flexion and pronation.

1 **Brachioradialis**

O: Lateral supracondylar ridge of humerus.

I: Lower outside surface of radius, proximal to styloid process.

A: Flexes elbow.

2 **Extensor carpi radialis longus**

O: Lateral supracondylar ridge of humerus.

I: Dorsal surface of base of second metacarpal.

A: Extends and abducts wrist.

3 **Extensor carpi radialis brevis**

O: Lateral epicondyle via common extensor tendon.

I: Dorsal surface of base of third metacarpal.

A: Extends and abducts wrist.

4 **Extensor carpi ulnaris**

O: Lateral epicondyle via common extensor tendon.

I: Base of fifth metacarpal.

A: Extends and adducts wrist.

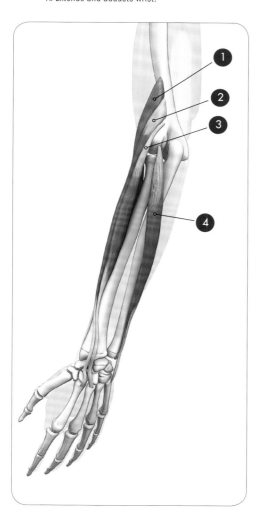

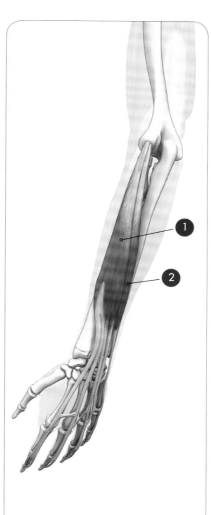

1 **Extensor digitorum**

O: Lateral epicondyle via common extensor tendon.

I: Dorsal surfaces of phalanges of all four fingers.

A: Extends fingers, synergizes finger abduction away from midline.

2 **Extensor digiti minimi**

O: Lateral epicondyle via common extensor tendon.

I: Combines with tendon of extensor digitorum to insert onto dorsum of little finger.

A: Extends little finger.

1 **Abductor pollicis longus**

O: Posterior surface of ulna and radius covering middle third of bones, interosseous membrane.

I: Lateral surface of first metacarpal.

A: Extends and abducts thumb, synergist of forearm supination and wrist flexion.

2 **Extensor pollicis brevis**

O: Posterior surface of distal radius, interosseous membrane.

I: Dorsal surface of base of proximal phalanx of thumb.

A: Extends thumb, synergizes wrist abduction.

3 **Extensor pollicis longus**

O: Posterior surface of middle third of ulna, interosseous membrane.

I: Dorsal surface at base of distal phalanx of thumb.

A: Extends thumb, synergizes wrist extension.

4 **Extensor indicis**

O: Posterior surface of distal ulna, interosseous membrane.

I: Dorsal aponeurosis of index finger, onto proximal phalanx.

A: Extends index finger.

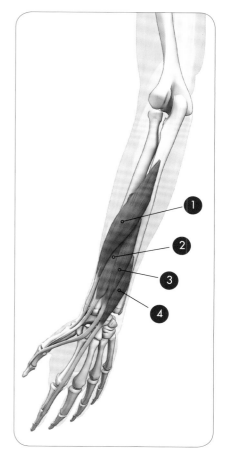

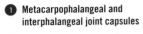

1 Metacarpophalangeal and
   interphalangeal joint capsules

2 Palmar radiocarpal and intercarpal ligaments

3 Palmar ulnocarpal ligament

1 Transverse metacarpal ligaments

2 Dorsal intercarpal ligaments

3 Dorsal radioulnar ligament

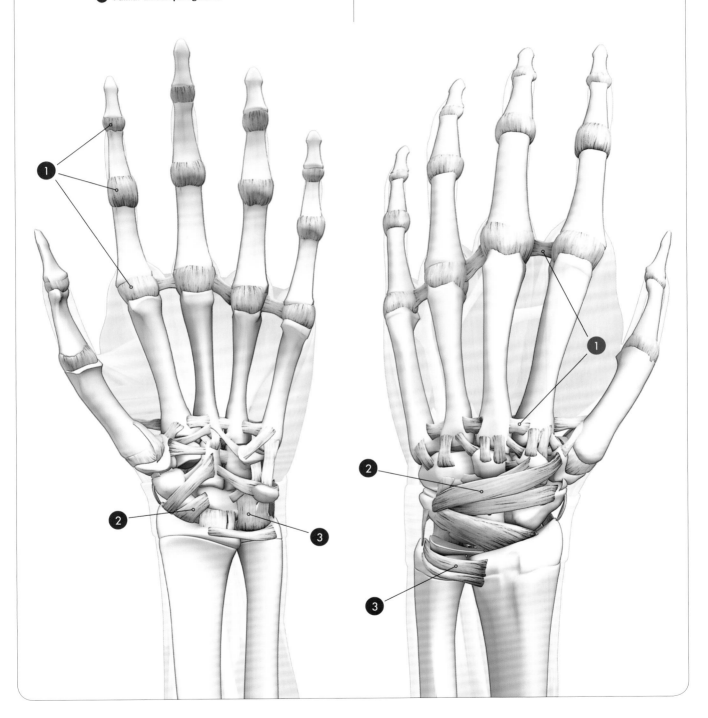

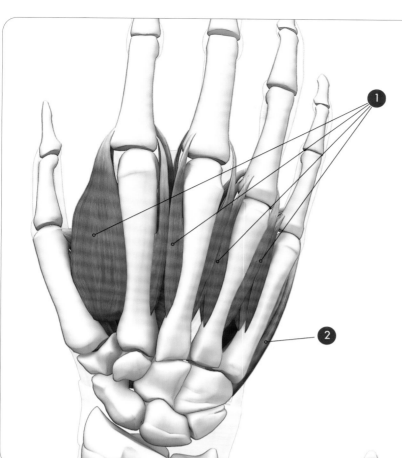

1 Dorsal interosseous muscles
O: Two heads, one from each side of adjacent metacarpal bones.
I: Base of proximal phalanx and dorsal digital expansions of fingers.
A: Abduct index and ring fingers away from middle finger, flex metacarpals, extend phalanges.

2 Abductor digiti minimi
O: Pisiform bone.
I: Ulnar side of proximal phalanx of little finger.
A: Abducts little finger.

1 Adductor pollicis
O: Palmar surface of capitate and trapezoid bones of the wrist, second and third metacarpals.
I: Base of proximal phalanx of thumb on ulnar side.
A: Adducts thumb.

2 Flexor pollicis brevis
O: Trapezium and capitate bones of wrist.
I: Base of proximal phalanx of thumb on radial side.
A: Flexes carpometacarpal and metacarpophalangeal joints of thumb, synergizes opposing thumb to little finger.

3 Abductor pollicis brevis
O: Trapezium and scaphoid bones of wrist, flexor retinaculum.
I: Base of proximal phalanx of thumb on radial side.
A: Abducts and moves thumb in palmar direction, synergizes opposing thumb to little finger.

4 Lumbrical muscles
O: Flexor digitorum profundus tendon.
I: Tendon of extensor digitorum.
A: Simultaneous flexion of metacarpophalangeal and extension of interphalangeal joints.

5 Flexor digiti minimi brevis
O: Hamate bone of wrist.
I: Base of proximal phalanx of little finger on ulnar side.
A: Flexes little finger.

6 Abductor digiti minimi

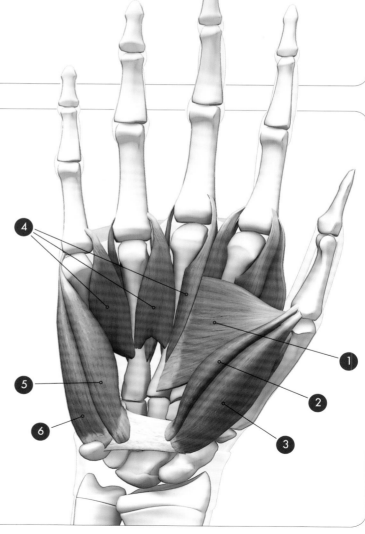

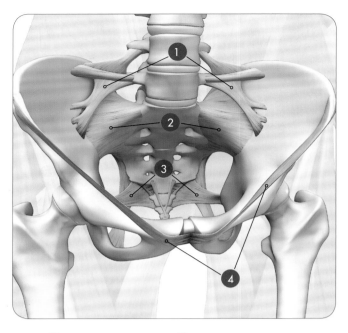

1 Iliolumbar ligament   3 Sacrospinous ligament

2 Sacroiliac ligament   4 Inguinal ligament

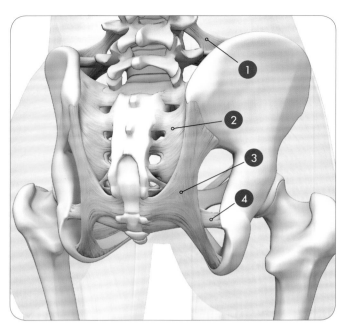

1 Iliolumbar ligament   3 Sacrotuberous ligament

2 Sacroiliac ligament   4 Sacrospinous ligament

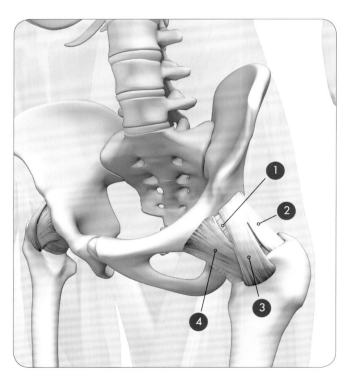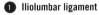

1 Zona orbicularis (hip capsule)   3 Anterior iliofemoral ligament

2 Lateral iliofemoral ligament   4 Pubofemoral ligament

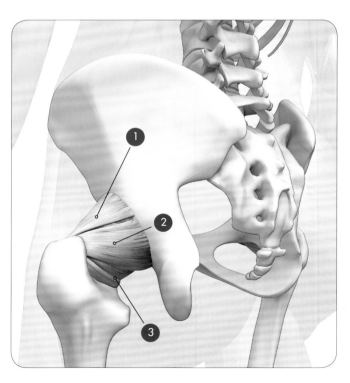

1 Lateral iliofemoral ligament   3 Zona orbicularis (hip capsule)

2 Ischiofemoral ligament

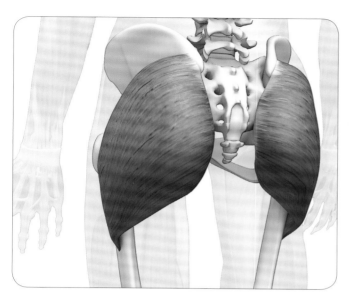

Gluteus maximus

O: Posterolateral surface of ilium and lateral surface of the sacrum.

I: Upper fibers onto iliotibial tract; lower fibers onto gluteal tuberosity.

A: Extends, externally rotates, and stabilizes hip.

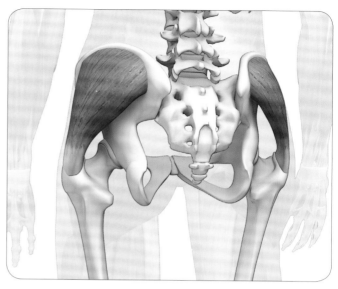

Gluteus medius

O: Outer surface of ilium.

I: Greater trochanter.

A: Abducts hip, anterior fibers internally rotate and flex hip, posterior fibers externally rotate and extend hip.

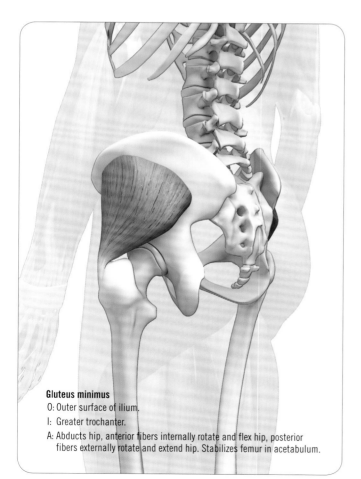

Gluteus minimus

O: Outer surface of ilium.

I: Greater trochanter.

A: Abducts hip, anterior fibers internally rotate and flex hip, posterior fibers externally rotate and extend hip. Stabilizes femur in acetabulum.

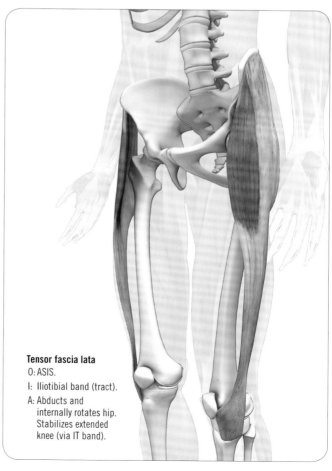

Tensor fascia lata

O: ASIS.

I: Iliotibial band (tract).

A: Abducts and internally rotates hip. Stabilizes extended knee (via IT band).

1 **Piriformis**
    O: Posterior surface of sacrum.
    I: Greater trochanter.
    A: Externally rotates, abducts, extends,
        and stabilizes hip.

2 **Superior gemellus**
    O: Ischial spine.
    I: Greater trochanter.
    A: Externally rotates and adducts hip.

3 **Obturator internus**
    O: Obturator membrane and ischium.
    I: Greater trochanter.
    A: Externally rotates and adducts hip.

4 **Inferior gemellus**
    O: Ischial tuberosity.
    I: Greater trochanter.
    A: Externally rotates and adducts hip.

5 **Quadratus femoris**
    O: Ischial tuberosity.
    I: Intertrochanteric crest.
    A: Externally rotates and adducts hip.

6 **Obturator externus**
    O: Obturator membrane and ischium.
    I: Greater trochanter.
    A: Externally rotates and adducts hip.

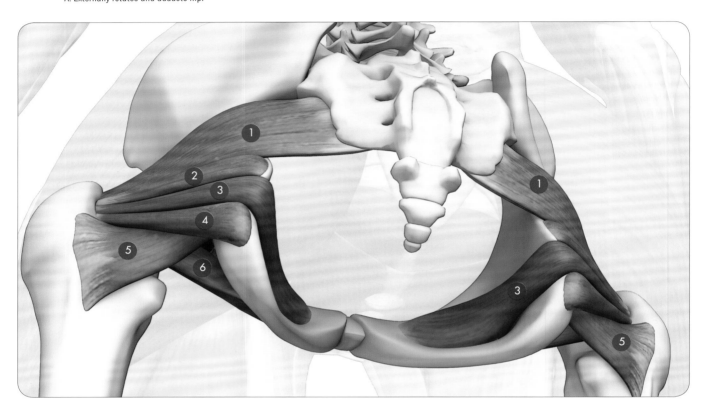

1 **Psoas major**
    O: T12-L4 vertebral bodies and discs.
    I: Lesser trochanter.
    A: Flexes and externally rotates hip,
        stabilizes lumbar spine.

2 **Iliacus**
    O: Inner surface of ilium.
    I: Lesser trochanter.
    A: Flexes and externally rotates hip,
        with psoas major tilts pelvis forward.

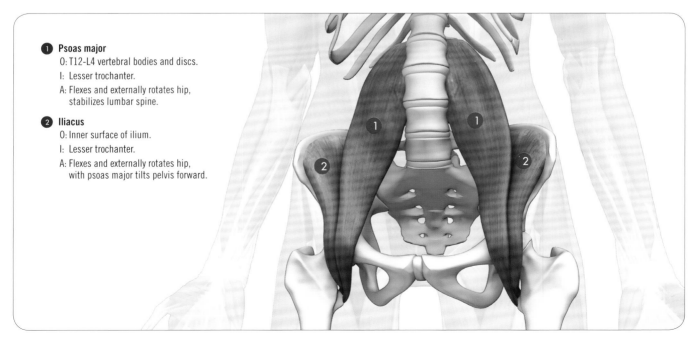

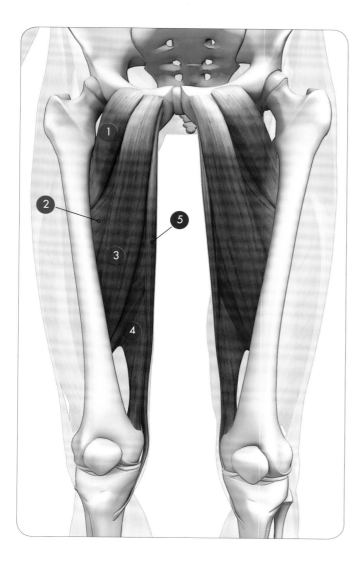

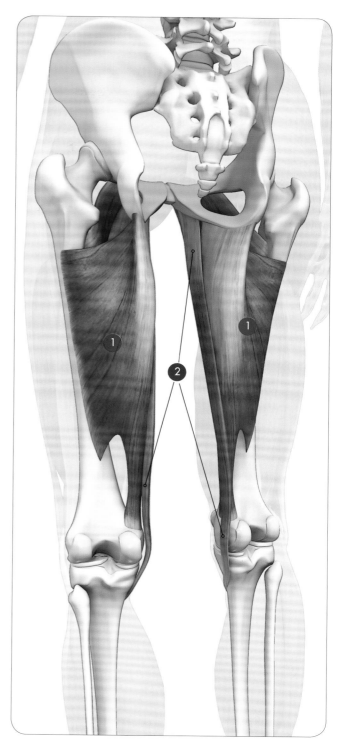

① **Pectineus**
O: Pubic bone.
I: Linea aspera of femur.
A: Adducts, externally rotates, and synergizes femur flexion.

② **Adductor brevis**
O: Pubic bone.
I: Linea aspera of femur.
A: Adducts and flexes femur, stabilizes pelvis.

③ **Adductor longus**
O: Pubic bone.
I: Linea aspera of femur.
A: Adducts and flexes femur, stabilizes pelvis.

④ **Adductor magnus**
O: Pubic bone and ischial tuberosity.
I: Linea aspera and medial epicondyle of femur.
A: Adducts, externally rotates, and extends femur.

⑤ **Gracilis**
O: Pubic bone.
I: Medial tibia.
A: Adducts and flexes hip, flexes and internally rotates knee.

① **Adductor magnus**

② **Gracilis**

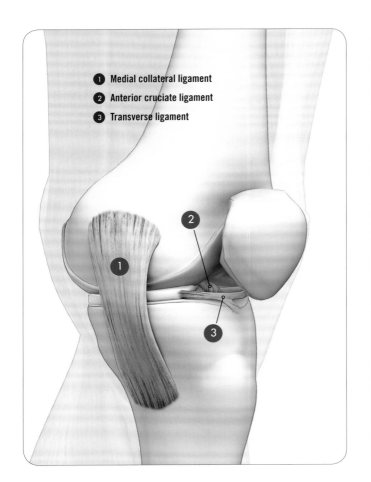

1 Medial collateral ligament
2 Anterior cruciate ligament
3 Transverse ligament

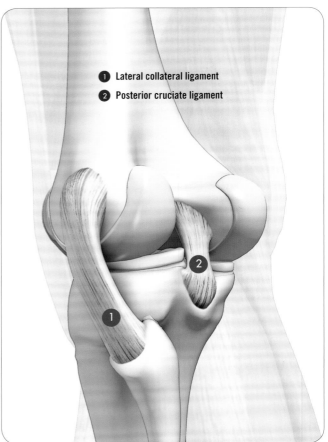

1 Lateral collateral ligament
2 Posterior cruciate ligament

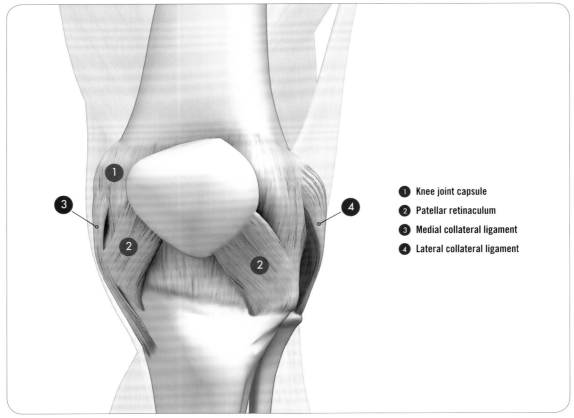

1 Knee joint capsule
2 Patellar retinaculum
3 Medial collateral ligament
4 Lateral collateral ligament

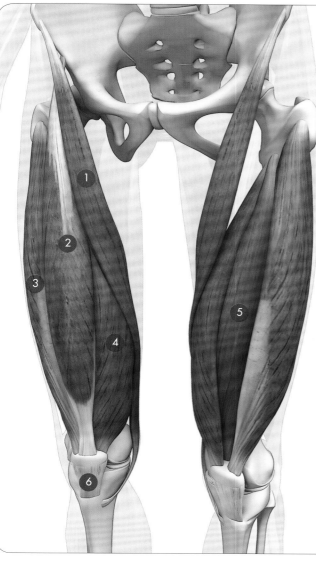

1 Sartorius
O: ASIS.
I: Pes anserinus of medial tibia.
A: Flexes, abducts, and externally rotates hip; flexes and internally rotates knee.

2 Rectus femoris
O: ASIS.
I: Anterior tibia via patellar tendon.
A: Flexes hip, tilts pelvis forward, extends knee.

3 Vastus lateralis
O: Lateral femur.
I: Anterior tibia via patellar tendon.
A: Extends knee.

4 Vastus medialis
O: Medial femur.
I: Anterior tibia via patellar tendon.
A: Extends knee.

5 Vastus intermedius
O: Anterior femur.
I: Anterior tibia via patellar tendon.
A: Extends knee.

6 Patellar tendon

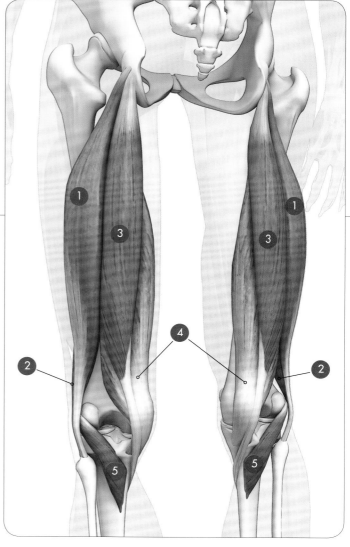

1 Biceps femoris long head
O: Ischial tuberosity.
I: Fibular head.
A: Extends hip, flexes and externally rotates knee.

2 Biceps femoris short head
O: Posterior surface of femur.
I: Fibular head.
A: Extends hip, flexes and externally rotates knee.

3 Semitendinosus
O: Ischial tuberosity.
I: Pes anserinus of medial tibia.
A: Extends hip, flexes and internally rotates knee.

4 Semimembranosus
O: Ischial tuberosity.
I: Back of medial tibial condyle.
A: Extends hip, flexes and internally rotates knee.

5 Popliteus
O: Lateral femoral condyle.
I: Posterior surface of tibia, below knee joint.
A: Flexes and internally rotates knee.

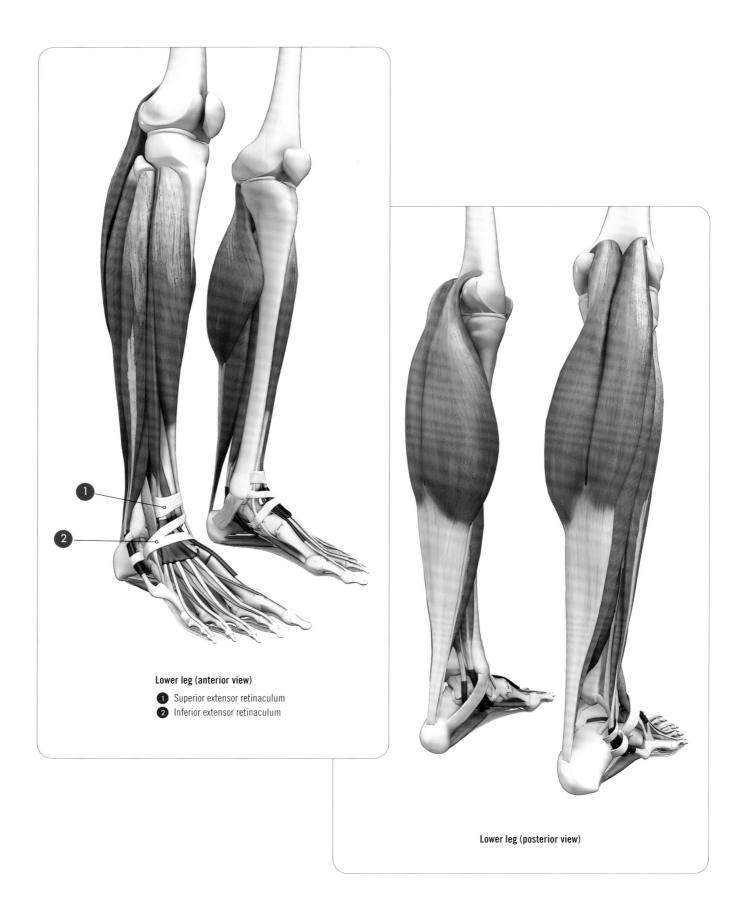

Lower leg (anterior view)

1. Superior extensor retinaculum
2. Inferior extensor retinaculum

Lower leg (posterior view)

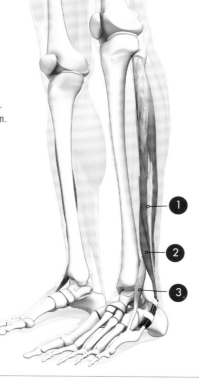

❶ Peroneus longus

O: Head and proximal two thirds of lateral fibula.

I: Base of first metacarpal and medial cuneiform.

A: Plantar flexes ankle and everts subtalar joint, supports transverse arch of foot.

❷ Peroneus brevis

O: Distal half of lateral surface of fibula, intermuscular membrane.

I: Base of fifth metatarsal.

A: Plantar flexes ankle and everts subtalar joint.

❸ Peroneus tertius

O: Front of distal fibula.

I: Base of fifth metatarsal.

A: Dorsiflexes ankle and everts subtalar joint.

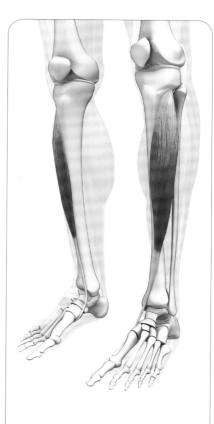

Tibialis anterior

O: Upper two thirds of anterior tibia and interosseous membrane.

I: Medial cuneiform, base of first metatarsal.

A: Dorsiflexes ankle, inverts subtalar joint.

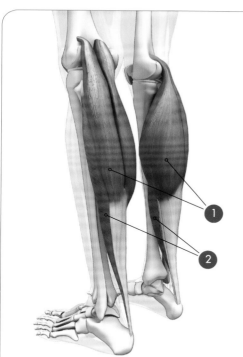

❶ Gastrocnemius

O: Medial head from medial epicondyle of femur; lateral head from lateral epicondyle.

I: Calcaneous via Achilles tendon.

A: Plantar flexes and inverts ankle, flexes knee.

❷ Soleus

O: Posterior surface of head and neck of fibula.

I: Calcaneous via Achilles tendon.

A: Plantar flexes ankle, inverts subtalar joint.

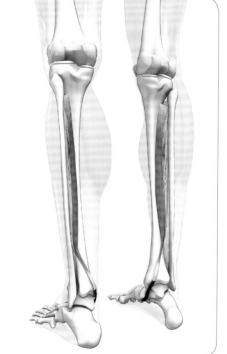

Tibialis posterior

O: Interosseous membrane between tibia and fibula.

I: Navicular, cuneiform bones, and second through fourth metatarsals.

A: Plantar flexes ankle, inverts subtalar joint, and supports longitudinal and transverse foot arches.

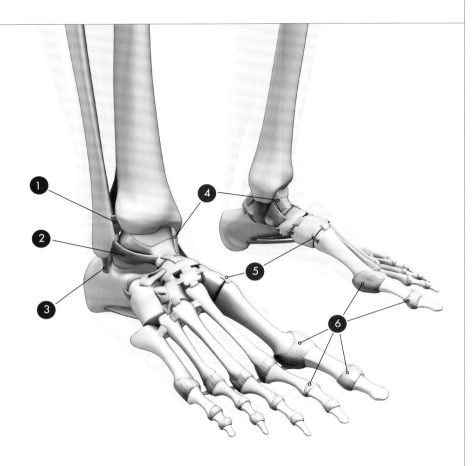

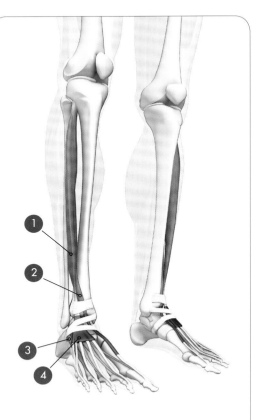

1. **Anterior tibiofibular ligament**
2. **Anterior talofibular ligament**
3. **Calcaneofibular ligament**
4. **Anterior tibiotalar ligament**
5. **Dorsal metatarsal ligaments**
6. **Interphalangeal joint capsules**

1. **Extensor digitorum longus**

   O: Lateral tibial condyle, fibular head, interosseous membrane.

   I: Dorsal aponeurosis and bases of the distal phalanges of second through fifth toes.

   A: Dorsiflexes ankle, everts subtalar joint, and extends metatarsophalangeal and interphalangeal joints of toes.

2. **Extensor hallucis longus**

   O: Medial surface of fibula, interosseous membrane.

   I: Dorsal aponeurosis and base of distal phalanx of big toe.

   A: Dorsiflexes ankle, everts subtalar joint, and extends big toe.

3. **Extensor digitorum brevis**

   O: Dorsal surface of calcaneous.

   I: Dorsal aponeurosis and bases of middle phalanges of second through fourth toes.

   A: Extends metatarsophalangeal and proximal interphalangeal joints of second through fourth toes.

4. **Extensor tendons sheath**

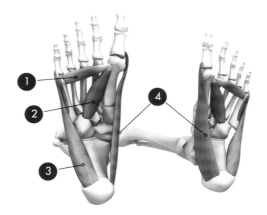

1 **Adductor hallucis (transverse head)**
   O: Metatarsophalangeal joints of third through fifth toes.
   I: Base of proximal phalanx of big toe via sesamoid.
   A: Adducts and flexes big toe, supports transverse foot arch.

2 **Adductor hallucis (oblique head)**
   O: Bases of second through fourth metatarsals, lateral cuneiform, and cuboid.
   I: Base of proximal phalanx of big toe via sesamoid.
   A: Adducts and flexes big toe, supports longitudinal foot arch.

3 **Abductor digiti minimi**
   O: Calcaneous, plantar aponeurosis.
   I: Base of proximal phalanx of little toe.
   A: Flexes metatarsophalangeal joint and abducts little toe, supports longitudinal foot arch.

4 **Abductor hallucis**
   O: Calcaneous, plantar aponeurosis.
   I: Base of proximal phalanx of big toe.
   A: Flexes and abducts big toe, supports longitudinal foot arch.

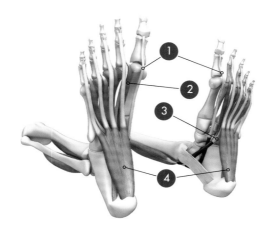

1 **Flexor hallucis longus**
   O: Posterior surface of fibula, interosseous membrane.
   I: Base of distal phalanx of big toe.
   A: Plantar flexes ankle, inverts subtalar joint, flexes big toe, supports longitudinal foot arch.

2 **Lumbrical muscles**
   O: Medial borders of flexor digitorum longus tendons.
   I: Dorsal aponeurosis of second through fifth toes.
   A: Flexes metatarsophalangeal and extends interphalangeal joints of second through fifth toes, adducts toes.

3 **Flexor digitorum longus**
   O: Posterior surface of tibia.
   I: Bases of distal phalanges of second through fifth toes.
   A: Plantar flexes ankle, inverts subtalar joint, plantar flexes toes.

4 **Flexor digitorum brevis**
   O: Calcaneous, plantar aponeurosis.
   I: Middle phalanges of second through fifth toes.
   A: Flexes toes, supports longitudinal foot arch.

1 Diaphragm

O: Lower margin of costal arch, posterior surface of xiphoid process of sternum, arcuate ligament of aorta, L1-3 vertebral bodies.

I: Central tendon.

A: Primary muscle of respiration, aids in compressing abdomen.

2 Intercostals

O: Internal intercostals from surface of upper margin of rib; external intercostals from lower margin of rib.

I: Internals insert on lower margin of next higher rib; externals insert on upper margin of next lower rib.

A: Internal intercostals lower ribs during exhalation; externals raise ribs during inhalation.

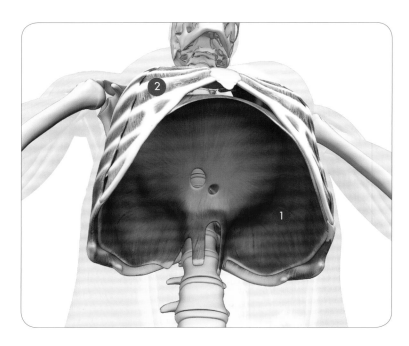

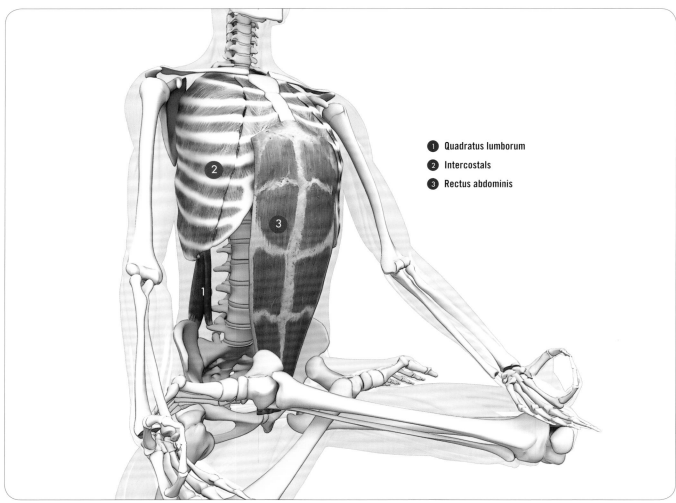

1 Quadratus lumborum

2 Intercostals

3 Rectus abdominis

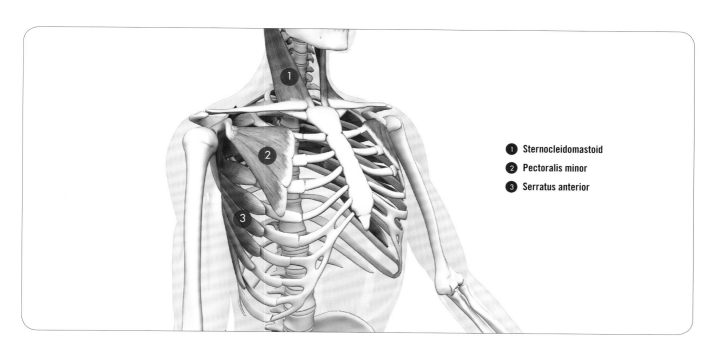

1 Sternocleidomastoid
2 Pectoralis minor
3 Serratus anterior

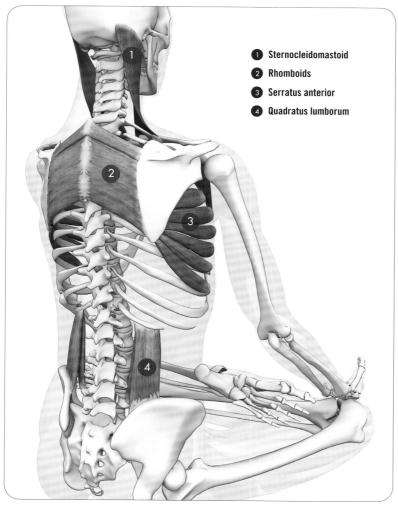

1 Sternocleidomastoid
2 Rhomboids
3 Serratus anterior
4 Quadratus lumborum

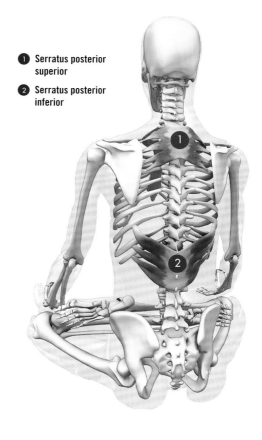

1 Serratus posterior superior
2 Serratus posterior inferior

INDEX OF MUSCLES
AND LIGAMENTS

GLOSSARY OF TERMS

Abduction Moving away from the midline.

Accessory muscles of breathing Muscles that attach to the ribcage and thorax that can be used to augment the action of the diaphragm for inhalation and exhalation. These include the rhomboids, pectorals, quadratus lumborum, sternocleidomastoid, and intercostals (among others).

Active insufficiency A condition in which a muscle is shortened or lengthened to a point where it can no longer effectively move a joint. For example, in Kurmasana the hips are fully flexed and so the psoas muscle is shortened to a point where it cannot effectively flex the hips further. At such times, other parts of the body must be used for leverage, such as the arms under the knees.

Adduction Moving toward the midline.

Agonist The muscle that contracts to produce a certain action about a joint (sometimes referred to as the prime mover). For example, the brachialis contracts to flex the elbow joint.

Alveoli Sac-like spherical structures with thin membrane-like walls through which gas exchange occurs in the lungs.

Anatomy The study of the structure of living things. Musculoskeletal anatomy studies the bones, ligaments, muscles, and tendons.

Antagonist The muscle that opposes the action of the agonist muscle and produces the opposite action about a joint. For example, the hamstrings are the antagonists to the quadriceps for extending the knee.

Anteversion Tilting forward.

Aponeurosis A fibrous thickening of fascia that forms the attachment for muscles. For example, the abdominal muscles attach to the linea alba, an aponeurotic thickening at the front of the abdomen.

Appendicular skeleton Composed of the shoulder (pectoral girdle) and upper extremities and pelvis and lower extremities.

Asana Sanskrit term for body position in yoga (yogasana).

Autonomic nervous system Part of the nervous system that functions largely unconsciously to control breathing, heart rate, blood pressure, digestion, perspiration, and other functions. It is divided into the sympathetic (fight or flight) and parasympathetic (rest and digest) nervous systems.

Axial skeleton Composed of the skull, spine, and ribcage.

Bandha Sanskrit term referring to binding, locking, or stabilizing. Co-activating muscle groups can be used to form bandhas in yoga postures.

Biomechanics The application of mechanical physics to the body. For example, contracting the biceps flexes the elbow joint.

Carpals The bones of the wrist, including the scaphoid, lunate, triquetrum, hamate, capitate, trapezoid, and trapezium.

Center of gravity The center of an object's weight distribution and at which point an object is in balance.

Center of gravity projection An extension of the force of gravity downward and away from the body. For example, in Warrior III the center of gravity is projected out through the arms and the back leg, balancing the pose.

Chakra Wheel-like centers or concentrations of energy within the subtle body. They may correspond to collections of nerves such as the lumbosacral plexus (for the first and second chakras).

Closed chain contraction/movement The origin of the muscle moves and the insertion remains stationary. For example, the psoas contracts to flex the trunk in Trikonasana.

Co-contraction/co-activation Simultaneously contracting agonist and antagonist muscles to stabilize a joint. For example, co-activating the peroneus longus and brevis and the tibialis posterior muscles stabilizes the ankle joint.

Core muscles Composed of the transversus abdominis, internal and external obliques, rectus abdominis, erector spinae, psoas, gluteus maximus, and pelvic diaphragm.

Drishti Sanskrit term for focus of vision or gaze.

Eccentric contraction The muscle generates tension (contracts) while lengthening.

Erector spinae The group of three deep back muscles that run parallel to the spinal column, including the spinalis, longissimus, and iliocostalis muscles.

Eversion Rotating the sole of the foot (via the ankle) away from the midline of the body. This is associated with pronation (internal rotation) of the forefoot.

Extension Joint movement that increases space and distance between skeletal segments, bringing them farther apart.

Facilitated stretching A powerful method of stretching in which the muscle is first taken out to its full length and then contracted for several moments. This stimulates the Golgi tendon organ and produces the "relaxation response," causing the muscle to relax and lengthen. It is also known as PNF.

Fascia Connective tissue that surrounds, separates, and binds muscles to each other. This can also form an aponeurosis for muscle attachment.

Flexion Joint movement that decreases space between skeletal segments and draws them closer together.

Floating ribs Five pairs of ribs that articulate posteriorly with the vertebrae and attach to the costal cartilage anteriorly.

Forefoot The region of the foot distal to the midfoot. It is composed of the metatarsal and phalangeal bones (and their corresponding joints). Motion includes toe flexion and extension and deepening of the foot arches.

Glenohumeral joint Ball and socket synovial joint where the head (ball) of the humerus articulates with the glenoid fossa (socket) of the scapula.

Golgi tendon organ A sensory receptor located at the muscle-tendon junction that detects changes in tension. This information is conveyed to the central nervous system, which then signals the muscle to relax, providing "slack" in the muscle. This protects against the tendon being torn from the bone. The Golgi tendon organ is central to PNF or facilitated stretching.

Hindfoot Typically refers to the calcaneous and talus bones. The joint for the hindfoot is the subtalar joint, which is responsible for everting and inverting the foot. For example, the hindfoot is inverted in the back leg in Warrior I.

Iliotibial tract Fibrous fascial structure that runs on the outside of the thigh and blends into the lateral portion of the knee capsule. This forms the attachment for the tensor fascia lata and part of the gluteus maximus muscles.

Impingement Narrowing or encroachment of the space between two bones. It can cause inflammation and pain. For example, a nerve root can become impinged by a herniated intervertebral disc. You can also have impingement between the humeral head and the acromion, causing pain in the shoulder.

Insertion The distal site where a muscle attaches to a bone (via a tendon), usually farther from the midline of the body and more mobile than the muscle origin at its opposite end.

Inversion Rotating the sole of the foot towards the midline of the body (turning it inward). This is associated with supination (external rotation) of the forefoot.

Isometric contraction The muscle generates tension but does not shorten, and the bones do not move.

Isotonic contraction The muscle shortens while maintaining constant tension through a range of motion.

Kriya Sanskrit term for action or activity.

Leverage Creating a mechanical advantage based on the length of the lever. For example, placing the hand on the outside of the foot in Parivrtta Trikonasana uses the length of the arm for leverage to turn the body.

Line of action A line through which forces act or are directed within the body. For example, there is a line of action extending from the tips of the fingers to the heel in Utthita Parsvakonasana.

Metacarpals The intermediate region of the hand between the carpus (wrist) and the fingers, i.e., the five bones of the palms of the hands.

Midfoot The intermediate region of the foot between the hindfoot and forefoot. It is composed of the navicular, the cuboid, and three cuneiform bones. Motion includes contribution to supination and pronation of the forefoot.

Mudra Sanskrit term for seal; similar to a bandha. It is often performed with the hands by bringing the fingertips together in a specific way. Other mudras are created by combining bandhas throughout the body.

Muscle spindle A sensory receptor within the muscle belly that detects changes in length and tension in the muscle. This information is conveyed to the central nervous system which can then signal the muscle to contract to resist stretching. This reflex protects against tearing the muscle.

Open chain contraction/movement The insertion of the muscle moves and the origin remains stationary. For example, the deltoids contract to lift the arms in Warrior II.

Origin The proximal site where a muscle attaches to a bone (via a tendon), usually closer to the midline of the body and less mobile than the muscle insertion on the bone at its opposite end.

Parivrtta Revolving, twisted, or turning version of a pose. For example, Parivrtta Trikonasana is the revolving version of Trikonasana (Triangle Pose).

Pelvic girdle The ilium, ischium, pubic bones, and pubic symphysis.

Physiology The study of the functional processes of living things. Most physiological processes take place unconsciously but can be influenced by the conscious mind. Examples include breathing and facilitated stretching.

PNF Proprioceptive neuromuscular facilitation. Also known as *facilitated stretching*. (See facilitated stretching.)

Posterior kinetic chain Composed of a group of interconnecting ligaments, tendons, and muscles on the back of the body. Includes the hamstrings, gluteus maximus, erector spinae, trapezius, latissimus, and posterior deltoids.

Pranayama Yogic art of controlling the breath.

Prime mover The muscle that contracts to directly produce a desired movement. For example, the quadriceps contracts to extend the knee joint. The term is sometimes used interchangeably with 'agonist muscle.'

Radial deviation Tilting the hand toward the index-finger side or away from the midline of the body.

Reciprocal inhibition A phenomenon whereby the brain signals an agonist muscle to contract, and a simultaneous inhibitory signal is sent to the antagonist muscle, causing it to relax. This physiological process takes place unconsciously.

Retroversion Tilting backward.

Rotation Joint movement around a longitudinal axis. For example, we externally rotate the humerus bones (longitudinal axis) to turn the palms to face up in Savasana.

Scapulohumeral rhythm Simultaneous movements at the glenohumeral and scapulothoracic joints that function together to abduct and flex the shoulders. For example, scapulohumeral rhythm takes place when we raise the arms overhead in Urdhva Hastasana.

Shoulder girdle The clavicles and scapulae.

Synergist A muscle that assists and fine-tunes the action of the agonist or prime mover. It can be used to produce the same action, although generally not as efficiently. For example, the pectineus muscle synergizes the psoas in flexing the hip joint.

True ribs Seven pairs of ribs that articulate posteriorly with the vertebrae and anteriorly with the sternum.

Ulnar deviation Tilting the hand toward the little-finger side or midline of the body.

SANSKRIT PRONUNCIATION AND POSE INDEX

Sanskrit	Pronunciation	Pages
Utthita Hasta Padangusthasana	[oo-tee-tah ha-sta pod-ang-goosh-TAHS-anna]	106
Urdhva Dhanurasana	[OORD-vah don-your-AHS-anna]	1, 8, 12, 19, 22, **76**, 84, 86, 106, 108
Urdhva Mukha Svanasana	[OORD-vah MOO-kah shvon-AHS-anna]	**47**, 58
Ustrasana	[oosh-TRAHS-anna]	13, 28, 38, **52**, 58, 106, 185
Virasana	[veer-AHS-anna]	62
Vrksasana	[vrik-SHAHS-anna]	106
Vrschikasana	[vrish-CHEE-kahs-anna]	**92**

Other Sanskrit Terms	Pronunciation	Pages
Asana	[AHS-anna]	——
Ashtanga	[UHSSH-TAWN-gah]	——
Bandha	[bahn-dah]	26
Chakra	[CHUHK-ruh]	45, 90
Drishti	[dr-ISH-tee]	4
Hatha	[huh-tuh]	1, 4
Jalandhara Bandha	[jah-lahn-DHA-rah bahn-dah]	——
Kriya	[kr-EE-yah]	——
Mudra	[MOO-drah]	——
Mula Bandha	[moo-lah bahn-dah]	43, 50, 57, 97, 128
Namasté	[nah-moss-te (*te* rhymes with *day*)]	142
Pranayama	[PRAH-nah-yama]	——
Susumna Nadi	[sue-SHOOM-nah NAH-dee]	124
Udyana Bandha	[oo-dee-YAH-nah BAHN-dah]	——
Ujjayi	[oo-jy (*jy* rhymes with *pie*)-ee]	——
Vinyasa	[vin-YAH-sah]	——
Yoga	[YO-gah]	——

ENGLISH POSE INDEX

CONTRIBUTORS

CHRIS MACIVOR—a self-taught computer expert and digital artist—is the Technical Director for Bandha Yoga and Illustrator of the bestselling series, *The Key Muscles of Yoga* and *The Key Poses of Yoga*. He is a graduate of Etobicoke School of the Arts, Sheridan College, and Seneca College. With a background in dance and traditional art, as well as computer graphics and animation, Chris considers himself to be equally artistic and technical in nature. Working with Dr. Long on the Scientific Keys book series, he has digitally reproduced the biomechanical perfection of the human body. With a keen eye for subtle lighting and a passion for excellence in his art, Chris successfully brings his imagery to life.

KURT LONG, BFA, is an award-winning fine artist and anatomical illustrator who contributed the front and back cover illustrations. He is a graduate of the University of Pennsylvania and has studied at the Pennsylvania Academy of Fine Arts and the Art Students League of New York. Kurt resides in Philadelphia with his wife and two sons. For information on commissions and to see more of his work, go to www.KurtLong.net.

STEWART THOMAS contributed the Sanskrit calligraphy and the special hand-painted border for the Bandha Yoga Codex. He is an award-winning artist, calligrapher, printmaker and designer. A graduate of Haverford College and the University of the Arts in Philadelphia, he serves as Creative Director of Florida's Eden, a regional alliance working for a sustainable future for North Florida, and produces art at his own Palmstone Studio (www.palmstone.com).

ERYN KIRKWOOD, MA, RYT 200, graduated from Carleton University with a Master's Degree in English Literature. She left a corporate career as Managing Editor at the Canadian Medical Association to dedicate her life to the study, practice, and teaching of yoga. Eryn is the Chief Editor at Bandha Yoga and maintains an award-winning Blog. She offers alignment-focused yoga classes in Ottawa, Canada, and can be reached at www.BarrhavenYoga.com.

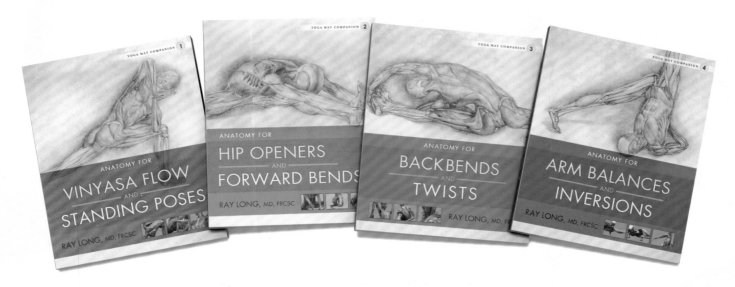

ALSO FROM BANDHA YOGA

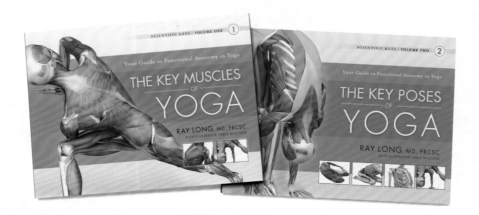

www.BandhaYoga.com